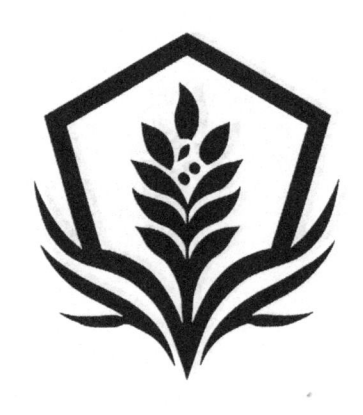

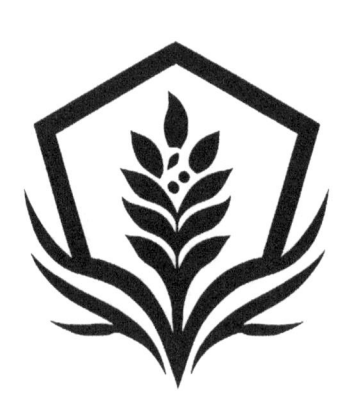

STOP!

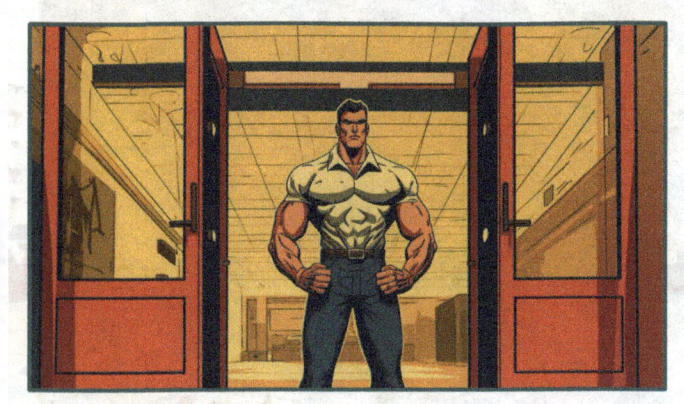

HAVE YOU READ THE PREVIOUS SPRING 2023 ISSUE OF RENEGADE HEALTH MAGAZINE YET?

The previous issue of Renegade Health Magazine contains 30 contributors specializing in fitness, nutrition, lifestyle, mindset, food preparation, general wellness, and more.

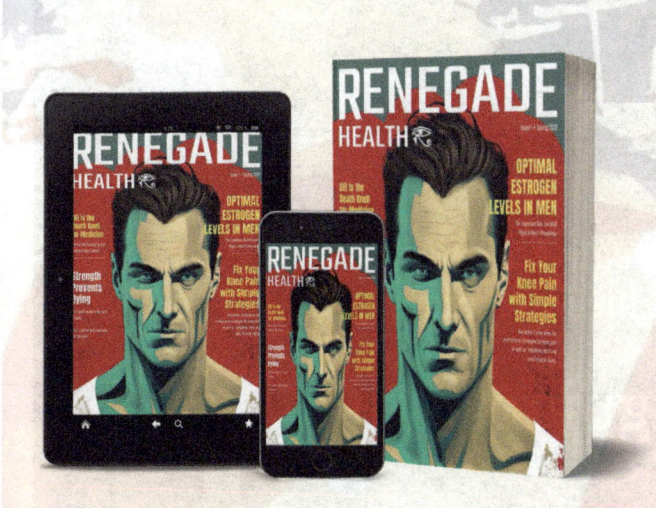

Here are just SOME of the Articles in the previous issue:

Physical Therapy

- *Fix Your Knee Pain with Simple Strategies* by Alexander Cortes
- *Restore Lost Range of Motion In Any Joint* by BowTied Kobra
- *Understanding Shoulder Impingement* by BowTied Bengal
- *Building Stronger, Denser Bones for Life* by Hybrid Athlete
- *The Site of the Pain Is Never the Source* by Alexandre Bernier

Weight Training

- *Strength Prevents Dying* by Marc Lobliner
- *Building a Legit Natural Physique* by Francis Melia

Medicine

- *My Diabetes Journey* by Benjamin Braddock
- *Diabetes Damages The Heart* by Brady Holmer
- *How to Avoid A Heart Attack* by Philip Ovadia

And MORE!

Get it at:
RenegadeHealthMagazine.com

The A.I. Art Master Guide

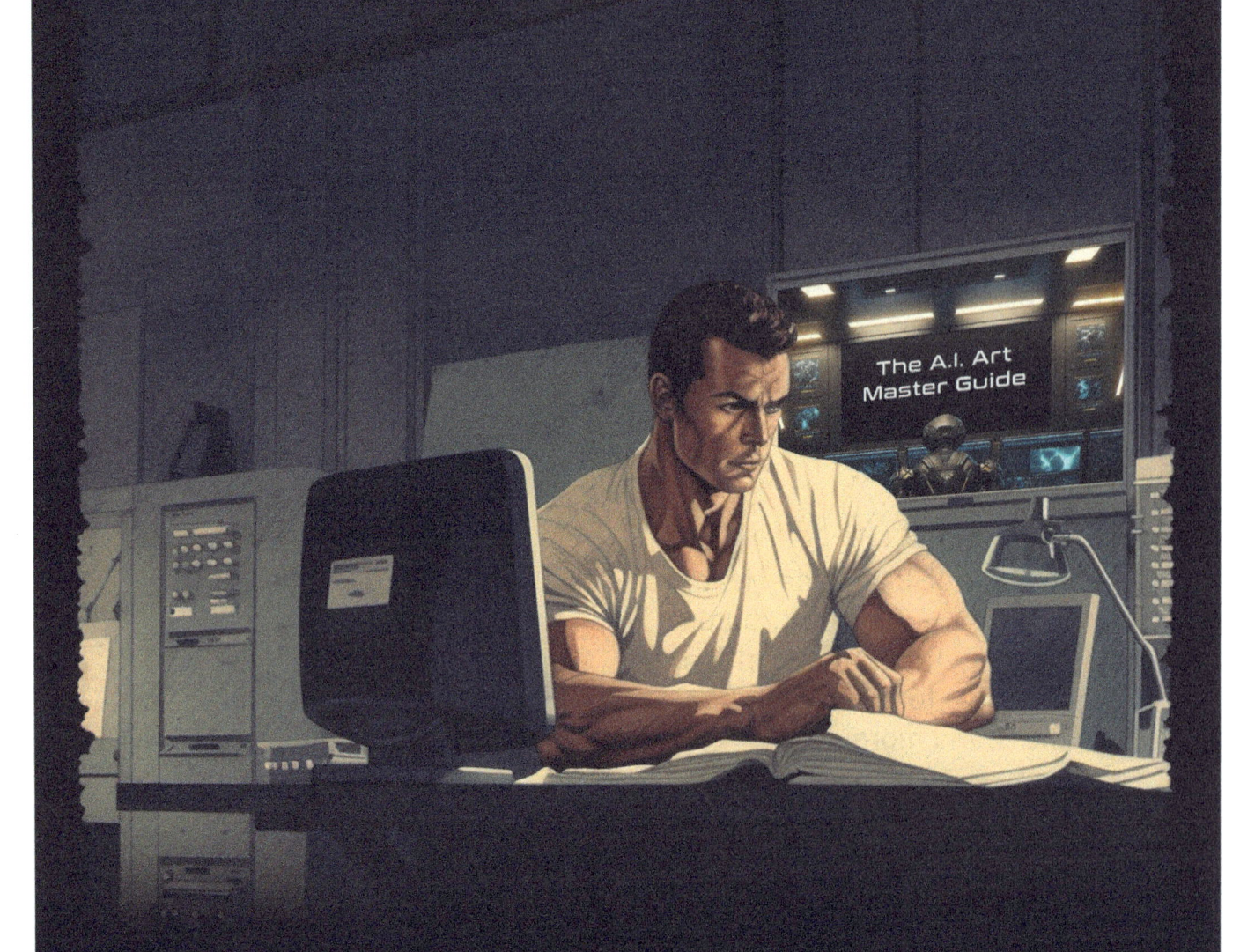

Learn how to create any
graphic you can imagine in seconds.

www.theaiartguide.com

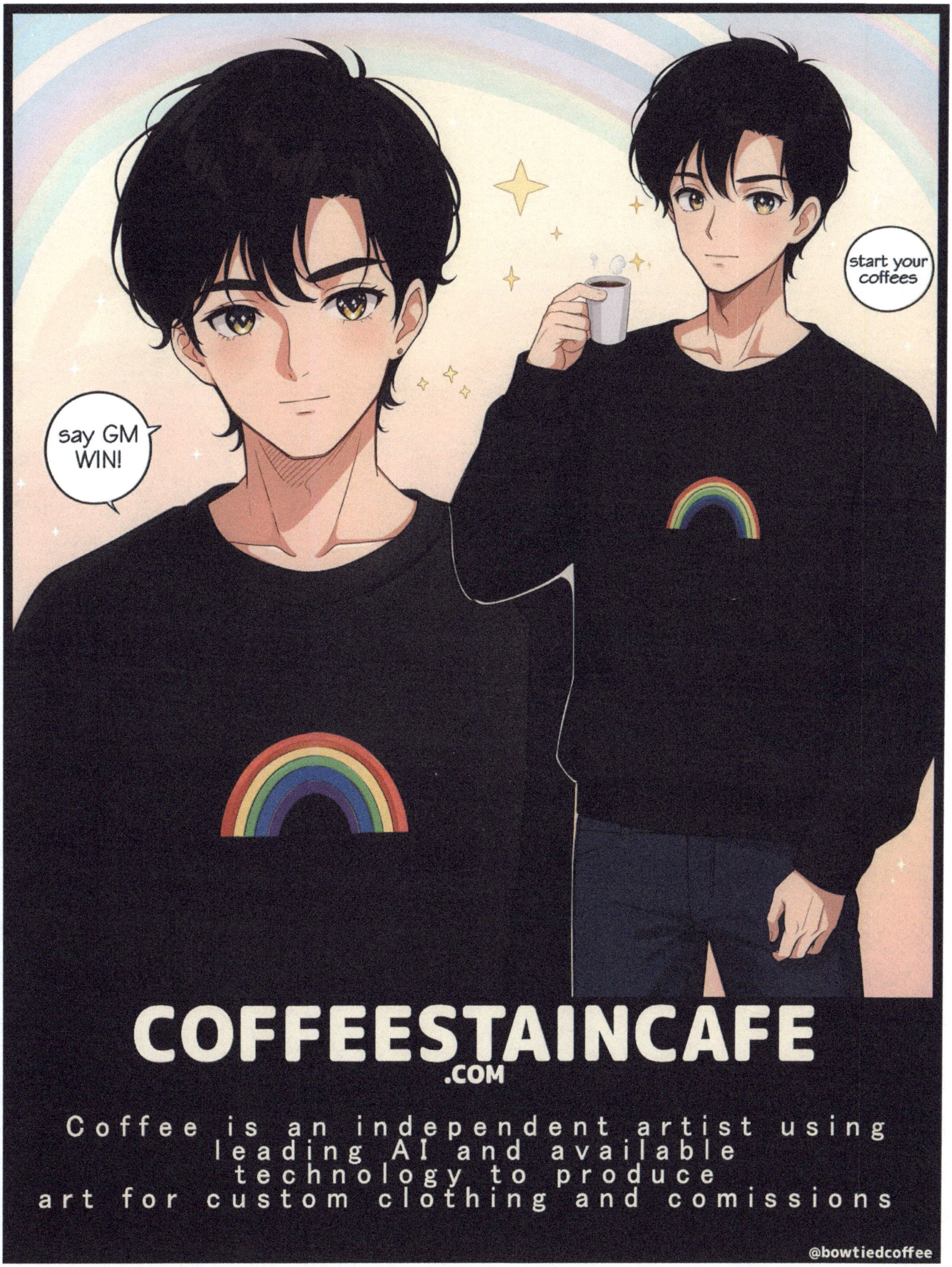
say GM WIN!
start your coffees
COFFEESTAINCAFE
.COM
Coffee is an independent artist using leading AI and available technology to produce art for custom clothing and comissions
@bowtiedcoffee

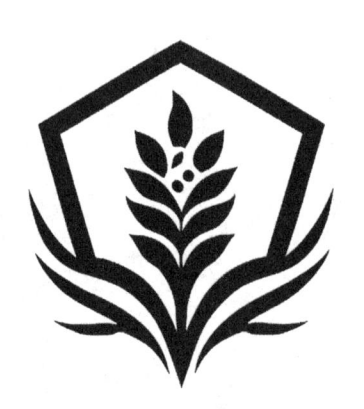

ISSUE 2 — SUMMER 2023

RENEGADE HEALTH

MOST people never take the first step towards becoming healthy. With your purchase of Renegade Health Magazine, you just did. Thank you for caring enough about your health to purchase this magazine.

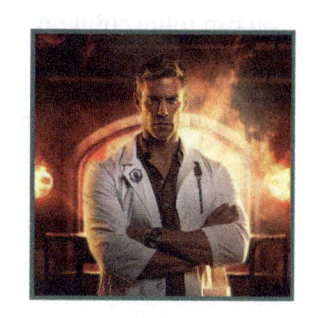

When I started RHM, it was a shot in the dark. I had no idea who, if anyone, would read almost 100 pages of dense health information. Frankly, I didn't care if the only people who bought a copy were myself and my mother. The health information space has been severely damaged by the last 3 years of Covid-19 propaganda. This magazine was a necessity. I consider it my duty to teach real health to as many people as possible.

Those of you who bought the first issue of Renegade Health Mag probably noticed it was nothing like the typical health magazines on the shelves. Instead of fulfilling their noble mission, they fill 100 pages with 50% advertisements, 40% celebrity gossip, and 10% useless advice. Have you ever wondered how they can afford to sell the magazine for $7? It's because they don't care who buys it; they've already cashed the checks from their biggest customers—advertising agencies.

There's nothing inherently wrong with advertising. In fact, it's the best way to get your product in front of the people who need your product the most. However, after the last 3 years, it's become clear the advertiser model is broken in the healthcare space. It's all government propaganda and Big Pharma crap.

Renegade Health Magazine chose to be different. You are our customer and our sole focus. We don't take advertisers. We rely solely on your support. Because of people like you, we are able to continue creating this magazine and sharing this valuable information.

Thank you.

Now I'm asking you to go one step further. Share it with someone. It can be your parents, friends, or a loved one. Post it on social media. Give us an honest review and let us know what we did well, as well as what we can improve on. Every little bit helps. And we appreciate it.

If you've got a creative suggestion to spread the message, we're all ears. I encourage you to email us at RenegadeHealthMag@proton.me.

For those of you interested in going one step further and contributing to Renegade Health Magazine, the door is always open. If you're a subject-matter-expert in some topic within the health field, we want to help you to share your knowledge to a larger audience. We have a contact page on our website at RenegadeHealthMagazine.com. Use it or email us directly.

Thank you for purchasing your copy of Renegade Health Magazine, and enjoy!

Doc Anarchy
@DoctorAnarchist

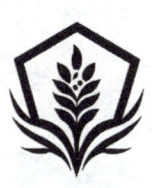

ISSUE 2　　　　　　　　　　　　　　　　　　　　　　　　　　　　　　　　　　　　SUMMER 2023

Doc Anarchy *is an expert at promoting health through lifestyle changes, rather than medications. He was an outspoken supporter of early treatment against Covid-19 and the author of* Killing Covid, *the definitive covid early treatment guideline. He is currently one of the top publishers in the Substack Health and Wellness category.*

You can follow him on Twitter at:
@DoctorAnarchist

And read his Substack at:
https://docanarchy.substack.com

Disclaimer

This magazine provides general information and discussions about health and related subjects. The information and other content provided in this magazine, or in any linked materials, are not intended and should not be construed as medical advice, nor is the information a substitute for professional medical expertise or treatment.

If you or any other person has a medical concern, you should consult with your health care provider or seek other professional medical treatment. Never disregard professional medical advice or delay in seeking it because of something that have read on this blog or in any linked materials. If you think you may have a medical emergency, call your doctor or emergency services immediately.

The opinions and views expressed in this magazine have no relation to those of any academic, hospital, health practice or other institution. The views expressed by individual authors in this magazine are their views, and should not be attributed to Renegade Health Magazine.

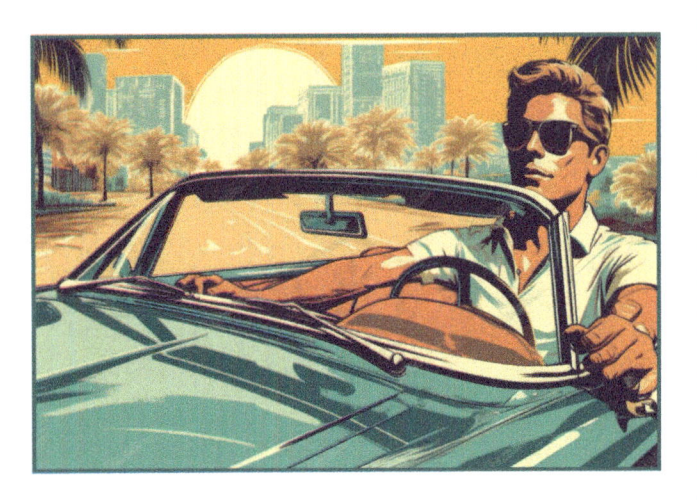

Renegade Health Magazine

Proven results. Competency over credentials.

Website:
RenegadeHealthMagazine.com

Twitter:
@RenHealthMag

Email:
RenegadeHealthMag@proton.me

Magazine Design, Layout, and Interior Artwork:
@BowTiedThinker | BowTiedThinker.com

Magazine Front Cover Artwork:
@BowTiedMaker | TheAIArtGuide.com

Magazine Rear Cover Artwork:
@BowTiedCoffee | CoffeeStainCafe.com

Copyright © 2023 Renegade Health Magazine

All rights reserved. No part of this publication may be reproduced, distributed, or transmitted in any form or by any means, including photocopying, recording, or other electronic or mechanical methods, without the prior written permission of the publisher, except in the case of brief quotations embodied in critical reviews and certain other noncommercial uses permitted by copyright law.

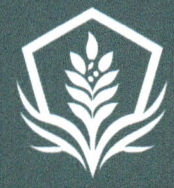

ISSUE 2 SUMMER 2023

IN THIS ISSUE:

Medicine
- Who Spiked Your Balls 11
- Modern Life Mitigation & Circadian Reset 14
- Should I See a Naturopathic Physician? 19
- Disc Herniation: To Cut, or Not to Cut? 22
- Mitochondria: The Missing Piece in Health Care 24
- How Medical Guidelines Work 27
- Serum, Moisturizer, and How to Use Them 29

Mental Health
- My Journey Through Drug Addiction 32
- Why Man Needs Emotion 36
- Your Daily Meditation Practice 38
- Zookeeping ADHD 41

Commentary
- Is Our Medical System Beyond Hope? 43
- Understanding Your Cost of Care 46
- The Bitcoin Cure 49
- What Is Value Based Care? 52
- Coercion Is Not Consent 54
- Optimal Nutrition For Preconception and Gestation 56
- Four Mistakes During Cycle Syncing and Menses 57
- Biting Into The Truth 59
- Crooked to Straight 63

Fitness
- The FleX Theory of Power 65
- Avoiding Back Pain From Deadlifts 71
- Breathe Your Way To Better Health 74
- Conquer Your Sleep Disorder: Part II 77
- Warning: The "Red Pill" is True (sort of) 79

Food
- Meet Your Protein Demands 83
- Take Control of Your Food Chain 86
- Get Prepared for The Cold and Flu Season 91
- The Principles of Regenerative Agriculture 94

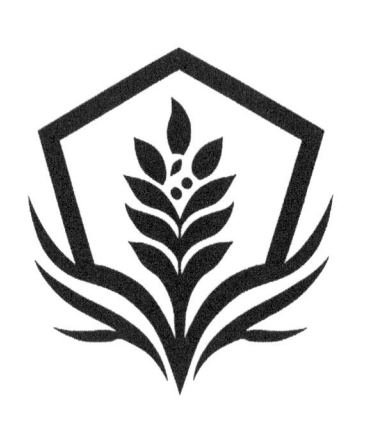

ISSUE 2 SUMMER 2023

Who Spiked Your Balls?

Dr. Lynn Fynn

LIVING through the past three years of continuous fear, ticker tapes of "cases" and death, unreasonable and ineffective policies, and misinformation-overload, much of the male population has unfortunately succumbed to taking a new genetic therapy that neither prevented infection nor mitigated spread of the etiological agent of Covid-19.

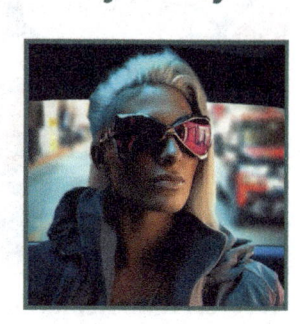

Many were required by their employers or wanted to travel, while others were forced by family to be able to visit with them. Both the therapy and the stress from constant information exhaustion certainly does not contribute to the overall health of the family jewels.

The most common complaint seen from those that took at least two of the Pfizer, Moderna, Janssen, or AZ injections is that they have not felt the same since. Though evidence of numerous chronic and debilitating diseases has "coincidentally" become common post-injection, including deadly outcomes, there are other issues that are less apparent as they aren't routinely tested. These may contribute to that feeling of "not normal."

Itai Gat, et al. studied such a phenomenon, particularly with mRNA technology, later published in the journal, Andrology, Covid-19 vaccination BNT162b2 temporarily impairs semen concentration and total motile count among semen donors.[1] Seeing as though the lipid nanoparticles used to carry the mRNA codons to the cells have been shown in the animal model to accumulate in the testis, it's not surprising that they would be affected by a highly inflammatory cationic lipid in addition to the production of a non-human protein at high concentrations, whereby eliciting an immune response that can attack those human cells programmed to produce it. This was a longitudinal study that demonstrated a deterioration of sperm count and motility for 3 months. This study was early following vaccine rollout and had not taken into consideration the long term effects of boosters and bivalents, which show a wider, dose-dependent toxicity profile.

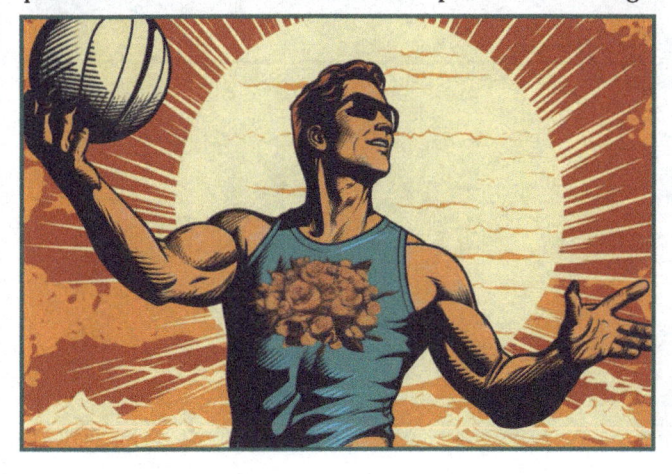

What is a man to do? Whether faced with fertility concerns or a potentially detrimental, premature drop in free testosterone, there is hope. Testosterone levels are assessed using a blood test. The cutoff for low testosterone differs between organizations, but most define it as a total testosterone level of <231–275 ng/dL. Testosterone levels should be assessed early in the morning (between 7–11 a.m.) when peak levels occur, and in a fasted state. Two separate low testosterone measurements (preferably four weeks apart) along with clinical signs and symptoms of low testosterone are needed to be diagnosed with low testosterone.

Some easily available supplements and pharmaceuticals can not only potentially return you to normal, but perhaps can help you as you age. First rule, no more Covid-19 vaccines. Secondly, See your doctor or Urologist. Unfortunately, many physicians are unaware of the effects of autoimmune mRNA damage, or the mechanisms involved; they should at least check your PSA, testosterone, blood chemistries and hematology. It's also not a terrible idea to shell out the extra money for a Cardiac MRI with gadolinium contrast to check for cardiac inflammation or other potential subclinical effects. Nothing is healthier than peace of mind.

The following are some potential treatments that may help you feel like yourself again.

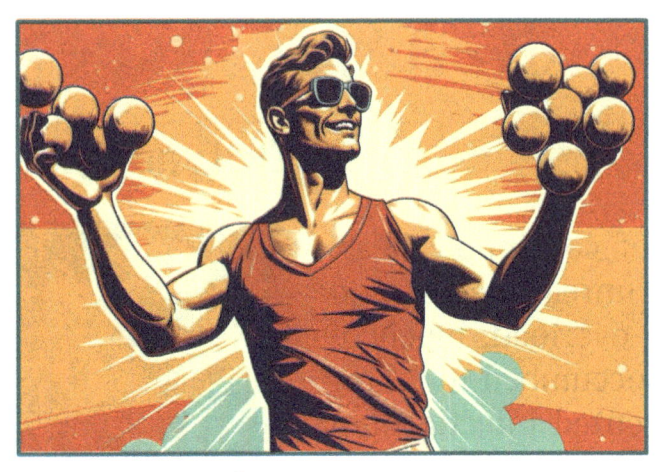

Testosterone Replacement

Though not an OTC supplement, there are many clinics that specialize in optimizing male hormones as they age. Testosterone is easily supplemented in a variety of treatments. These include bi-weekly injections, oral supplements, nasal gel, topical cream, transdermal patch, or implantable pellets every 3–4 months. TRT does not come without potential adverse events. Discuss risks with your physician. Supplementing testosterone in this manner will lower your natural ability to produce. A way around this is to dose testosterone/nandrolone 2:1 every 4 days with the addition of a dose of hCG (human chorionic gonadotropin) the day before your injection). Discuss the optimal dosing with your physician.

Clomiphene Citrate

A selective estrogen receptor modulator, clomiphene citrate, can boost testosterone up to 250% when taking 25 mg a day. By blocking those receptors, negative feedback is shut down, allowing testosterone production to flourish. This is an often overlooked yet excellent alternative to TRT without shutting down natural production.

Vitamin D

Effect of vitamin D supplementation on testosterone levels in men, showed a significant increase in total and free testosterone compared to placebo.[2] Doses of 4000 IU a day can have a significant impact. Do take 100 mcg of K2 (MK-7) for every 4000 IU D3 you take. This prevents your bones from being robbed of calcium.

Testofen/Fenugreek

Glycosides of Fenugreek, marketed under the name Testofen, have shown androgenic and anabolic effects in males. A meta-analysis of published literature from Cochrane, PubMed, Scopus, Web of Science and Google Scholar were examined, and the conclusion suggests that the supplement had significant effects on total serum testosterone suggesting that it can be used to increase total testosterone levels.

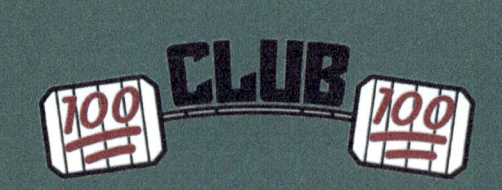

What Is The 100 Club?

Many of the Personal Success Stories in this issue were written by members of the 100 Club.

The 100 Club is a Twitter community valuing health, fitness, working hard, and being good citizens. There is no single leader, rather a group of like-minded members who support each other to improve their lives. They help people set goals and overcome difficult challenges in their daily lives.

You won't only find gym bros in the 100 Club. There are veterans, doctors, fitness coaches, and average people with incredible health transformations. They support charity, currently hosting fundraisers to donate to the PTSD Foundation of America.

There are no rules, fees, or inauguration to join the 100 Club. You must simply set a goal and follow the ethos of improving yourself by setting and achieving individual goals. The 100 Club will provide you with the motivation and resources you need to accomplish your goals, whether that means losing weight, gaining muscle, quitting smoking, or just improving your health overall.

If you want to meet new friends, learn about fitness and nutrition, and join a supportive online community, consider joining the 100 Club.

If interested, reach out to @100club100 on Twitter.

Zinc

Zinc deficiency can hinder testosterone production. Like magnesium, zinc is lost through sweat. Therefore, athletes and other people who sweat a lot are more likely to be deficient. Although dietary zinc is mostly found in animal products, zinc-rich foods include some grains and nuts (pardon the pun) and can also be taken as a supplement.[3]

Spike Neutralization

It took years to fine-tune the protocol for post-vaccination damage. Though one cannot claim the all-encompassing "detox" one can neutralize some effects of persistent spike production from the mRNA codons in different parts of the body. The most comprehensive that I've found that can still be followed compliantly is the FLCCC post vaccine protocol.[4]

Overall, patients have reported a notable improvement in overall health since post vaccine symptoms presented. Many supplements known to contribute to men's health, such as nattokinase for circulation, and magnesium, are included in this protocol.

Exercise

Whether aerobic exercise, high-intensity interval training, or resistance training—they all increase testosterone, especially when included as part of a lifestyle intervention to reduce body weight. Cutting out the sugar and starch along with intermittent fasting can all contribute to lowering body weight and stimulating testosterone production. Exercise may also improve the effectiveness of TRT. Bariatric surgery is another effective method for increasing testosterone levels in obese men. Exercise, along with quality sleep, are a man's best friend.

Conclusion

Whichever route you choose to support natural testosterone production or replace when you can no longer produce, studies have proven better overall health and longevity. If you examine the link between serum testosterone, free testosterone and DHT and the all-cause mortality risk of 16,451 community-dwelling older men from Perth in Western Australia in 2013 Yeap et al. paper, it should be obvious that the third quartile of all these serum values, is where you want your androgen levels to be, if you intend to live to see your 90th birthday.

Sources

1. https://pubmed.ncbi.nlm.nih.gov/35713410/
2. https://pubmed.ncbi.nlm.nih.gov/21154195/
3. https://ods.od.nih.gov/factsheets/Zinc-HealthProfessional/
4. https://covid19criticalcare.com/wp-content/uploads/2023/02/I-RECOVER-Post-Vaccine-Summary-1.pdf

Works Cited

- Ramasamy, R., Fisher, E. S., & Schlegel, P. N. (2012). Testosterone replacement and prostate cancer. Indian journal of urology: IJU: journal of the Urological Society of India, 28(2), 123.
- Yeap, B. B., Alfonso, H., Chubb, S. P., Handelsman, D. J., Hankey, G. J., Almeida, O. P., ... & Flicker, L. (2013). In Older Men an Optimal Plasma Testosterone Is Associated With Reduced All-Cause Mortality and Higher Dihydrotestosterone With Reduced Ischemic Heart Disease Mortality, While Estradiol Levels Do Not Predict Mortality.
- Perry III, H. M., Miller, D. K., Patrick, P., & Morley, J. E. (2000). Testosterone and leptin in older African-American men: relationship to age, strength, function, and season. Metabolism, 49(8), 1085-1091.
- Rodriguez, A., Muller, D. C., Metter, E. J., Maggio, M., Harman, S. M., Blackman, M. R., & Andres, R. (2007). Aging, androgens, and the metabolic syndrome in a longitudinal study of aging. Journal of Clinical Endocrinology & Metabolism, 92(9), 3568-3572.
- Rohrmann, S., Nelson, W. G., Rifai, N., Brown, T. R., Dobs, A., Kanarek, N., ... & Platz, E. A. (2007). Serum estrogen, but not testosterone, levels differ between black and white men in a nationally representative sample of Americans. Journal of Clinical Endocrinology & Metabolism, 92(7), 2519-2525.
- Traish, A. M., Miner, M. M., Morgentaler, A., & Zitzmann, M. (2011). Testosterone deficiency. The American journal of medicine, 124(7), 578-587.
- Vermeulen, A., Verdonck, L., & Kaufman, J. M. (1999). A critical evaluation of simple methods for the estimation of free testosterone in serum. Journal of Clinical Endocrinology & Metabolism, 84(10), 3666-3672.
- Xu, L., Au Yeung, S. L., Kavikondala, S., Leung, G. M., & Schooling, C. M. (2014). Testosterone concentrations in young healthy US versus Chinese men. American Journal of Human Biology, 26(1), 99-102.

Dr. Lynn Fynn *is is an MD with primary focus on Infectious Disease with an extensive background in Reproductive Endocrinology. She is a scientific writer for AFLDS and founding member of Global Covid Summit (https://globalcovidsummit.org/) and DeMed and has been at the forefront of early treatment since the start of the pandemic in addition to analyzing the shortfalls and dangers of mRNA injections as well as Remdesivir, Paxlovid and Molnupiravir.*

You can follow her on Twitter at:
@Fynnderella1

ISSUE 2 SUMMER 2023

Modern Life Mitigation & Circadian Reset

BH3

> **I HAVE** been blabbering about light for about a decade, way before most people knew what blue light was. The Blue Light Diet name was kind of cool, not trendy. I've been telling you about light forever because your body is a quantum machine. In a quantum machine, physics rules chemistry.

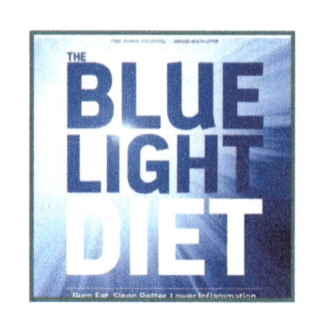

Light comes before diet and exercise. Yet, so many doctors and diet/exercise gurus totally ignore this fact when talking to patients and clients. I developed the Blue Light Diet protocol to fill in that gap.

I know your time is valuable and there are a lot of other good articles in this issue. Even the woke people at Harvard now tell you about the dangers of blue light, so I'm not going to make you read a million words here. I must, however, give you the surface level basics and action steps.[1] I promise your reading will be worth it. This article will tell you what one of your biggest health problems is and then give you the solutions.

The number one health issue you probably face today is modern life. Increasing population density augments the bad health effects of modern life.

How Is Modern Life Your Biggest Bad Health Threat?
Modern life inverts the way nature built you to live. AI contest the biggest health concern in modern life is bad lighting.

Instead of bright days filled with sunlight and dark nights filled with stars and moonlight, we are living and working mostly indoors. This gives you constant artificially lit but relatively dark days and chronic artificially lit, bright nights.

Some main health problems with the wrong kind of light or light at the wrong time include the following:

Retina & Opsin Damage
Most just think of the retina as part of your eye, but it is really an extension of your brain. Parts of it, like intrinsically photosensitive retinal ganglion cells, sense, and process light as information and relay it to your brain. This works like an orbiting moon or satellite that provides a direct superhighway of information to your brain's main control center, keeping time for and operating almost every system in your body.

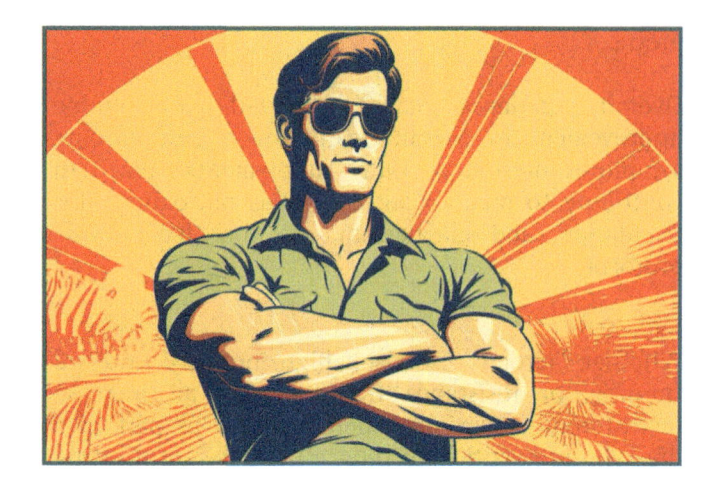

You also have these light sensing proteins called opsins found in your skin that sense changes in your light environment and make decisions based on that information.[2] You can think of them as eyes in your skin.

In nature, you never find blue light without red light. Blue light has higher energy photons which create more free radicals and is very stimulating. Red and infrared light is more regenerative and repairs some of the damage that blue light creates.[3] A problem is that most artificial light is severely lacking in red and infrared light and loaded with blue light. This artificially produced blue light gets to wage war on your retina and opsins day after day and night after night.

Circadian Rhythm Disruption
Your days are too dark, and your nights are too bright, and this creates chaos in your bodies internal clock, accelerating disease creation. I cannot make it any simpler. Over millions of years life has evolved to work

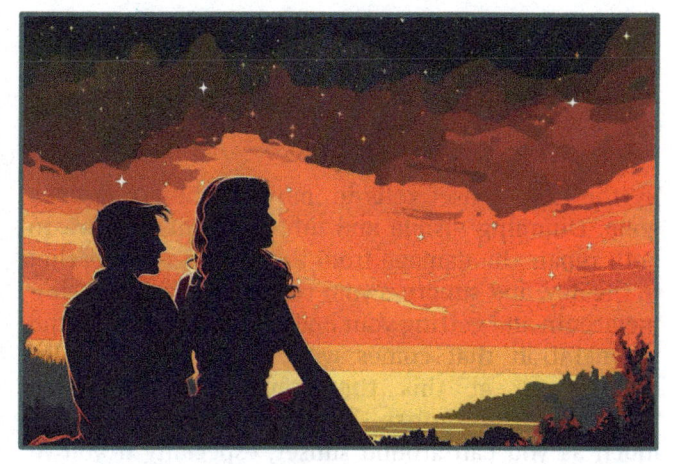

on a predictable rhythm governed by relatively predictable light and dark cycles. In just the last hundred or so years, modern life has learned how to turn night into day with the flick of a switch. This moved much of its day into the relative darkness of artificially lit indoor living. Dark days hurt you just as much as bright nights hurt you.[4,5] You must reverse this back to how nature built you to operate.

Lack of Sun
We already know the sun can predict stock market outcomes, but here's the even crazier thing, it can predict health outcomes too.[6] Unfortunately, your dermatologist is turning you into a lifelong money machine for the medical establishment. Despite what they say, the truth is that if you get more sun, you get less deadly cancers. Furthermore, other diseases take much longer to progress.[7] Get more sun. It is as simple as that. And if you get sunburn, you need more sun, not less. You wouldn't get sunburn much if you were living outside all day long according to how you were designed by nature or god. Sunlight is food for your mitochondria. It lowers stress, makes you feel naturally high, and creates energy inside of you by making electrons jump by way of Einstein's photoelectric effect.

Flicker
Think of watching light through a ceiling fan. It creates a quick on and off blinking effect. That is what flicker is and most types of artificial lighting have flicker whereas the sun and moon do not flicker. Flicker is usually undetectable with your eye and can be created by the electronics in LED lighting, light dimmers or even plugging a light into the AC power grid. Artificial flicker has been shown to cause all sorts of problems, including inducing migraines and other neurological and physiological effects.[8]

So how do you fix the problem of modern light and life?

Move out of big cities.

And if you can't move, you must mitigate to reverse the modernity in your life, which starts with creating bright days and dark nights as best you can.

Whether you can move or not, there are two steps to this Blue Light Diet modern mitigation protocol.

The first is a circadian reset to jumpstart your system and get it back into the natural rhythm it has probably been missing for years. The second is your own ongoing modern life mitigation protocol.

The Blue Light Diet Modern Circadian Rhythm Reset
There are a couple great studies out of the circadian research department at the University of Colorado Boulder.[9] Essentially what they showed was that you can totally reset your circadian rhythm in about a week. They achieved this by leaving the big city and going camping out in the wilderness. What they found was people living a modern lifestyle could reset their body clock to match the natural solar seasonal light cycle in their local environment with a week of camping.

If you can go camping for a week, or even a weekend, do it!

I understand most people probably can't get up and go camping for a week, so I've put together a circadian reset protocol for you that will simulate the camping experience as best as possible.

In order to do this we have to focus on light/dark, air, grounding/magnetism and food timing.

Light
Wake up with the sunrise and wind down with the sunset.

You want bright days and dark nights. The brightest mornings possible. Dark mornings predispose you to cancer and disease. This is one of the reasons daylight savings time is so bad for people.[10] You want to be outside during the day as much as you possibly can. Working in the shade or on a balcony is fine. Being outside is key because it exposes you to both changing wavelengths of sunlight and changing brightness of sunlight. Before modern life, the default way of living was outdoor bright light all day long. Now our days are too dark, and our health is suffering because of it.

If you cannot be outside all day, you need to take multiple sun breaks and expose yourself to bright light.

While inside during the day, try to be near an open

window and use bright incandescent or halogen bulbs with a color temperature of around 3000k. You could put together a little light bank of four bulbs or so and have them close to your workspace.

When you take your sun breaks, try to get sun on as much of your bare skin as possible. Much of the fear mongering over the sun and melanoma is nonsense. But don't be stupid and fry yourself—burning will cause damage.[11] Use logic and reason and get sun at a rate according to your skin type and what you think you can handle. Build your solar callus first and remember that early morning sun has a greater percentage of red and infrared light, which acts as nature's sunscreen to protect you from the stronger UV light later in the midday.[12]

⇒ First Exposure (Sunrise)
Sunlight around sunrise is nature's red light therapy machine, coffee, hormone regulator and sunscreen all wrapped up into one package. It syncs all your body clocks and sets your circadian rhythm, feeds your mitochondria breakfast, shuts down melatonin, boosts cortisol, and preps your skin for the stronger sunlight yet to come. Try your best to get up and see the sunrise through unfiltered eyes each morning. The big key to this period is the quick transition from dark to brighter light. If you get up before sunrise, wear a good pair of orange or red lens blue light blocking glasses. Do not see screen light before sunlight. Stay out as long as you can, minimum 15 minutes. You do not have to stare at the sunrise or even see it (it is more therapeutic if you can see it), just get outside or stick your head out of your window at that time.

⇒ Second Exposure
Around mid-morning, depending on what season it is and where you are in the world, UVA sunlight starts to increase in power. Among other things, UVA creates energy in your body by making electrons jump through Einstein's photoelectric effect, stimulates nitric oxide production, lowers blood pressure, and starts to round up some hormones. You want to get this sunlight in your eyes and on as much skin as possible. You can use the DMINDER App or local UV index to get a rough estimate when this period occurs.[13] You can consider a UVI of 2 to be the time to get outside for this period.

⇒ Third Exposure
Depending on where you are in the world, UVB starts to really emerge around 10am and peaks at solar noon. Use the Dminder or a weather app to determine when solar noon is in your exact location. This new UVB wavelength not only stimulates more melanin creation, but also interacts with your skin to create vitamin D and optimize your immune system. Ideally you stay out at this time until you receive your MED or minimal erythemal dose of UVB filled sunlight. You achieve this dose when your skin just turns the slightest bit pink or darker.

⇒ Fourth Exposure (Sunset)
By the time sunset rolls in, most of the UV light is gone. Dimming visible and infrared light is there to both repair the damage from the stronger sun earlier in the day, and suppress your cortisol while increasing melatonin and getting your body ready for the rest and regeneration that comes with darkness. The color temperature at this time reverts to the same temperature at sunrise. You want to be outside as much as you can around sunset, especially if you've been in the stronger sun earlier in the day. The biggest key to this period is letting your eyes and skin sense the relatively quick transition from light to dark.

⇒ Darkness
In nature, after sunset, infrared light never goes away. You are getting very faint starlight as well as moonlight, which is mostly an altered spectrum of reflected sunlight at nighttime. Your goal is to mimic this as much as possible once the sun sets. Get yourself a pair of blue and green light blocking glasses that actually work.[14] Use candlelight or fire. There are special red light bulbs you can use at night.[15] You have to make sure these aren't too bright, as bright enough red light can disrupt circadian rhythm. Ideally, light bulbs at night are placed at ground level and not overhead. Consider clothing or pajamas to be your nighttime sunscreen. Clothing can block artificial light from triggering photoreceptors in your skin and disrupting circadian rhythm locally.[16] Use filters for tech or TV screens.[17] There are also two computer programs you can use to reduce blue light and flicker on your screens. Iris costs a little bit and F.lux is free.[18,19] If you're in a big city, even with all your lights off there still is a huge afterglow which makes an unnaturally bright night sky. Use black out curtains and a sleep mask.[20] The only problem with blackout curtains or a sleep mask is that the morning light is too dark. You miss that gradual brightening. So mitigate appropriately and train yourself to get up a little before sunrise. Finally, turn off all electronics and unplug all lights in your bedroom. If for some reason you must have something on in your bedroom, cover the light with a piece of black electrical tape.

⇒ nnEMF
I don't have time to go into it in this article because it's a big rabbit hole, but nnEMF stands for Non Native Electro Magnetic Frequencies. This is all the invisible energy floating in the sky from man made devices like radio signals, Wi-Fi, and cell phones. nnEMF is a form of light, so you want to treat it just like you treat light and darkness. If you have to use it and be exposed to it, it's best to use it in the daytime when the natural

EMF is stronger as well. At night, you want to avoid it, just like you do artificial light as much as possible. Get it out of your bedroom! Measure with an EMF meter and block or turn off the nnEMF sources. I have a good source for EMF meters and blockers and anything else I mentioned here on my Amazon recommendations page.[21]

Air/Temperature
Indoor air pollution can be way worse for health than the air outside![22] While doing this circadian rhythm reset, you'll be outside a lot more in your local environment. While this is a good thing, you also want to keep some windows open at all times in your house, in addition to using a good air filter. Modern heating and air conditioning can also be a circadian rhythm disruptor.[23] Be reasonable. Extreme hot or cold is not good, no matter what it's like in your local environment. In general, it's better to be colder than hotter, especially in your bedroom at night. Wear more clothes or use more blankets if you are cold. Another big reason for keeping a window open, besides letting full spectrum sunlight into your house, is Co2. Co2 tends to be abnormally high indoors. Go to Amazon and get a cheap Co2 meter and measure your indoor environment. Average CO2 outside is 400 ppm but can be much higher indoors, which accelerates health problems. This begins to be a concern once you get above 500 ppm.[24] Ideally, you want your indoor CO2 readings to be as close as possible to the outdoor average of around 400 ppm.

Grounding/Magnetism
Think about your daily life. You wear shoes with rubber soles, and you sleep in an insulated house, probably on at least the second floor and sometimes in huge high rise buildings. You have disconnected yourself from the Earth. Furthermore, you likely have no Earth-to-skin contact, which contributes to many health issues.

When you are out in the wilderness doing a circadian reset, you are more connected directly to the Earth through electron and magnetic field connection! The Earth has a slightly net negative charge to it. It also has a magnetic field that tends to be larger and more stable during the night than the day.[25,26] The health benefits of bare skin-to-Earth contact, also known as grounding or earthing, are established but not well known by the public. The overall anti-inflammatory effects of grounding yourself to the Earth is my favorite benefit.[27] Your body and circadian rhythm are also both subtly influenced by magnetic field connection and dichotomy.[28,29]

In your modern circadian reset, you want to mimic this close connection to the Earth as much and as long as you can. When you are outside, try to be grounded. Go barefoot on the grass or the beach etc. When you are inside, you can use something called a "grounding mat" that is designed to bring Earth electrons to you indoors.

The problem with these is that some of them plug into the wall which can introduce different harmonics and dirty electricity to your mat. I use a grounding mat but I buy the extension cord and spike that sticks directly into the ground outside instead of an electrical outlet in your wall.[30]

Another useful tool is called a Magnetico sleep pad.[31] You put it under your bed and it produces a strong static magnetic field that helps to create that day/night magnetic field dichotomy. It's also good for nnEMF mitigation and anyone who sleeps indoors (more hypoxic) and higher up from the ground.

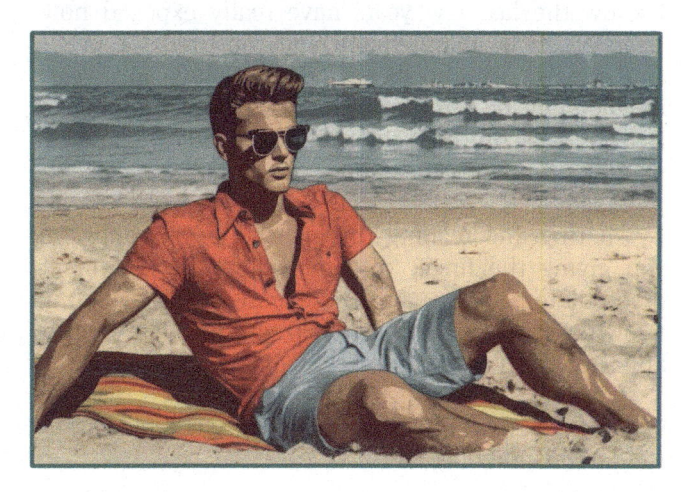

Food Timing
Light is the main focus of this article so I'm not going to comment about food too much except to mention two points. Food is a peripheral circadian clock setter.[32] It can reinforce or disrupt your circadian rhythm.[33] In order to support your circadian rhythm, you ideally want to eat soon after you wake up and also limit or stop any eating after the sun sets.[34] Your ideal goal should be to eat outside to allow the light in your food to interact with the light in your local environment.[35]

Eat more seafood. Seafood has lots of properly positioned DHA.[36] DHA is food for your circadian machinery because your retina is loaded with DHA and it helps keep your main circadian clock, the SCN, on time.[37] DHA is able to use its electron clouds to capture light photons and essentially turn them into an electrical signal.[38] You can kind of think of DHA as a molecule that lets you decode some of the wireless communication from the sun.

This food section can simply be broken down into eat more seafood and eat it when the sun is out.

Ongoing Modern Life Mitigation

After you have given a circadian reset including all of the above steps your best shot for one or two weeks, what do you do next?

Over the last week or two, you should have found your own rhythm. Your life should be a little less modern. Now take what worked for you in each area and make it a habit. You don't have to be as extreme, but in each of the area's above, try to get as close to nature as YOU possibly can for your current situation. Move out of the big city and if you can't, hack and mitigate each area as best you can.

That's it. You've got the general outline on how to reverse or mitigate modern life. Now you just have to commit to it.

I know the last few years have really exposed how science can be manipulated and censored for profit and power. People like you who buy and read independent research and publications like Renegade Health Magazine are the counterstrike to scientific manipulation and censorship.

By sharing and reading this magazine, not only are you giving the finger to the medical establishment manipulators, but you are also gaining knowledge only a few possess. This will help you improve your health and the health of those you care about.

That's the benefit of being out on the edge and not in the establishment center.

Out on the edge you see all kinds of things you can't see from the center.
Big, undreamed-of things-the people on the edge see them first.

Kurt Vonnegut

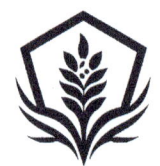

BH3 *teaches how circadian rhythm disruption from artificial light and lack of sun causes hidden health problems.*

You can follow him on Twitter at:
@BlueLightDiet

And see his Website at:
https://www.bluelightdiet.com

Sources

1. https://www.health.harvard.edu/staying-healthy/blue-light-has-a-dark-side
2. https://www.ncbi.nlm.nih.gov/pmc/articles/PMC7674233/
3. https://pubmed.ncbi.nlm.nih.gov/30825600/
4. https://www.ncbi.nlm.nih.gov/pmc/articles/PMC4632990/
5. https://www.ncbi.nlm.nih.gov/pmc/articles/PMC5454613/
6. https://www.milesfranklin.com/seasonal-affective-disorder/
7. https://www.ncbi.nlm.nih.gov/pmc/articles/PMC7400257/
8. https://www.ncbi.nlm.nih.gov/pmc/articles/PMC4038456/
9. https://www.cell.com/current-biology/fulltext/S0960-9822(13)00764-1
10. https://twitter.com/bluelightdiet/status/1504489036848664580
11. https://www.ncbi.nlm.nih.gov/pmc/articles/PMC3730314/
12. https://docanarchy.substack.com/p/prepare-for-sunlight-season
13. https://www.epa.gov/sites/default/files/documents/uviguide.pdf
14. https://www.bluelightdiet.com/blog/topfiveblueblockers
15. http://www.bluelightdiet.coom/links
16. https://twitter.com/bluelightdiet/status/1648680513832361984
17. http://www.lowbluelights.com
18. http://www.bluelightdetox.com/iris
19. http://www.justgetflux.com
20. http://www.bluelightdetox.com/manta
21. http://www.bluelightdiet.com/links
22. https://pubmed.ncbi.nlm.nih.gov/30202344/
23. https://www.ncbi.nlm.nih.gov/pmc/articles/PMC3427038/
24. https://www.ncbi.nlm.nih.gov/pmc/articles/PMC3548274/
25. https://web.ua.es/docivis/magnet/earths_magnetic_field2.html
26. https://earth-planets-space.springeropen.com/counter/pdf/10.1186/s40623-022-01656-9.pdf
27. https://www.ncbi.nlm.nih.gov/pmc/articles/PMC10105021/
28. https://www.nature.com/articles/458948f
29. https://twitter.com/bluelightdiet/status/1629203821502271499
30. http://www.bluelightdiet.com/links
31. https://magneticosleep.com/about-magnetism/scientific-validation/
32. https://www.ncbi.nlm.nih.gov/pmc/articles/PMC7182033/
33. https://twitter.com/bluelightdiet/status/1598333537417043968
34. https://twitter.com/bluelightdiet/status/1610317040937476096
35. https://twitter.com/bluelightdiet/status/1639255976581685250
36. https://twitter.com/bluelightdiet/status/1562269024859394048
37. https://www.ncbi.nlm.nih.gov/pmc/articles/PMC7601701/#:~:text=Of%20all%20the%20tissues%20in,phospholipids%20is%20DHA%20%5B1%5D.
38. https://pubmed.ncbi.nlm.nih.gov/23206328/

ISSUE 2 — SUMMER 2023

Should I See a Naturopathic Physician?

Dr. Alan Bradford, NMD

A RECENT poll conducted by Rasmussen Reports indicates that almost one third of Americans believe that public health officials have been lying to the public.[1] Polling from Gallup in 2021 showed a persistent decline in trust and confidence in doctors, with similar levels to poll results from 2002.[2]

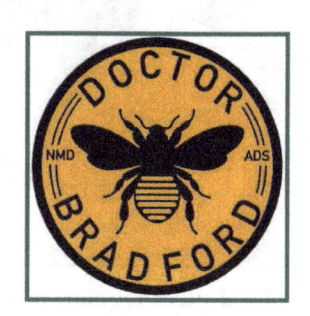

As our country becomes increasingly distrustful of the traditional western medical system, more than ever people are searching for alternatives. Enter the profession of the Naturopathic Physician.

There's a chance you may be scratching your head wondering what this is. Or maybe you think a Naturopathic Physician just recommends that you rub essential oils on everything. As of March 2023, only 23 states have licensing and registration laws in place for Naturopathic Physicians. From the American Association of Naturopathic Physicians' website: "In these jurisdictions, naturopathic doctors are required to graduate from accredited four-year residential naturopathic medical programs and pass an extensive postdoctoral board examination (NPLEX) in order to receive a license or registration."[3]

Scope of practice varies in each licensed state, but can include services such as ordering lab work and diagnostic imaging, prescribing medications (including controlled substances), administering IV therapy, and delivering babies. In 13 of these licensed states, a Naturopathic Physician is recognized as a primary care physician. Some may joke that the designation "ND" stands for "Not a Doctor." Believe it or not, in some situations this may be correct! There are folks out there who took a few online courses to become a "naturopath", but never graduated from a medical program or had any real life clinical experience. So be careful.

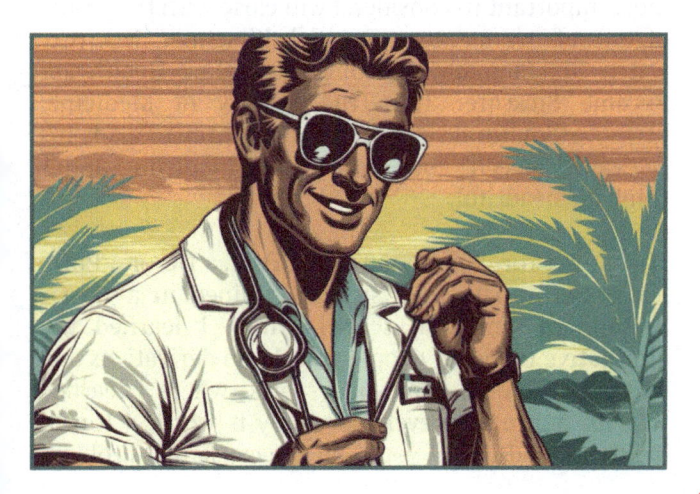

Legal and licensing information aside, I want to share three reasons why you may benefit from seeing a Naturopathic Physician.

1. My doctor tells me "everything is fine" but I feel like hot garbage.
2. I know I need to eat better, but I need help
3. All my doctor will do is prescribe medicine. There's got to be another way.

My Doctor Tells Me "Everything Is Fine" But I Feel Like Hot Garbage

A Naturopathic Physician approaches patient care from an entirely different paradigm. This is perhaps best summed up in a quote from one of my dear mentors, the late Dr. James Sensenig, ND. He told me one time: "There is no cure for the common cold. The cold is the cure." Dr. Sensenig unfortunately passed away December 1, 2019, right before the world went mad over a cold virus. I have no doubt he has turned over multiple times in his grave over the last three years.

In addition to approaching a patient with the philosophy of "do no harm", a Naturopathic Physician is trained in the mindset of "treat the whole patient (mind, body, spirit)", "prevention is the best cure", and "the healing power of nature." These foundational principles shape recommendations and generally result in excellent patient outcomes. A Naturopathic Physician worth his or her salt will be an expert in the functional interpretation of lab work. This means going beyond "normal values" reported by the lab, looking for patterns that may reveal digestive dysfunction, inflammation, or brewing issues with blood sugar regulation.

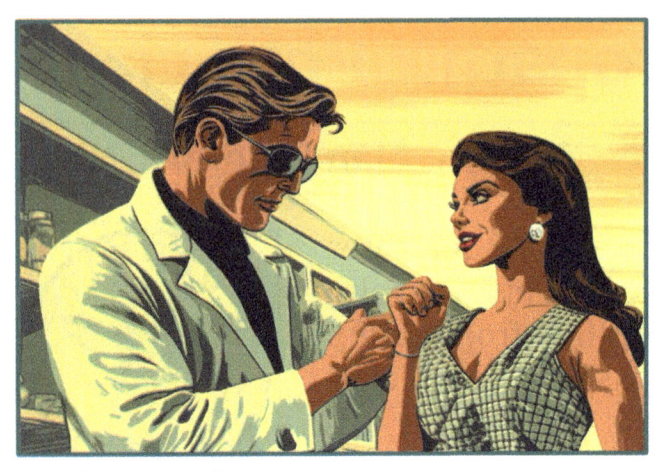

I cannot tell you how many times I've sat with a patient and told them things their other doctors never noticed in their lab work. One patient in particular came to me with a pile of labs from the past several years. As I thumbed through them, it was very clear that she had diabetes. Looking up from the papers, I casually asked her, "how long have you been diabetic?" She stared back at me, eyes like saucers. "Um...what do you mean? Nobody told me I was diabetic." If your doctor has been running basic lab work on you for years and telling you that "everything looks normal", you may want to consult with a Naturopathic Physician.

I Know I Need To Eat Better, But I Need Help

You don't know what you don't know, and I can tell you: allopathic physicians don't know nutrition. Traditional medical education does an abysmal job teaching medical students about nutrition. From a 2015 article on the American Medical Association website:

"Modern medicine maintains the importance of proper nutrition, yet on average, U.S. medical schools only offer 19.6 hours of nutrition education across four years of medical education...This corresponds to less than 1 percent of estimated total lecture hours. Moreover, the majority of this educational content relates to biochemistry, not diets or practical, food-related decision-making."[4]

I may be wrong, but I can't imagine things have improved since 2015.

Contrast this with the curriculum at an accredited Naturopathic medical school, where "students complete an average of 155 classroom hours of nutrition education."[5] That's at least 8x the amount compared to an MD or DO. No wonder all your allopathic doctor has to offer is the rote advice of "eat better." They may refer you to a dietitian, where you'll likely get further talking points that align with USDA-approved dietary advice. (I know how dietitians are trained; I completed an undergraduate degree in Human Nutrition, where many of my colleagues went on to become dietitians.) If you're struggling to make dietary changes, you may want to consult with a Naturopathic Physician.

All My Doctor Will Do Is Prescribe Medicine. There's Got To Be Another Way.

You've heard the phrase, "If all you have is a hammer, everything is a nail." In the digital age, the prescription pad has largely been replaced with electronic orders. Have no doubt, the digital prescription pad is still whipped out fast enough to make Doc Holiday blush. According to most recently available data from the CDC, 40% of adults over 65 years old are taking 5 or more prescriptions per day (compared to 14% in 1994). And nearly 20% of adults 45–65 years old are doing the same.[6]

I believe there is a time and place for everything, and in some situations pharmaceutical intervention may be appropriate. In the early 1990s, Dr. Jared Zeff, ND collaborated with a small group of Naturopathic Physicians on a project that culminated in the creation of the "Therapeutic Order of Naturopathic Medicine".[7] This is a set of guiding principles which directs decision-making in patient care. It consists of seven different levels of care, starting with "low-force" interventions and culminating in "high-force" interventions, which may include surgery. It's not until you get to the fifth level of the Therapeutic Order that you find "synthetic symptom relief,", which would include pharmaceutical drugs. Prior to this, a Naturopathic Physician may recommend dietary and lifestyle changes, strategies for stress management, botanical medicines, acupuncture, and more. If you're tired of trying to restore health with modern chemical concoctions (and unhappy with the results!), you may want to consult with a Naturopathic Physician.

There are plenty of other reasons to consult with a Naturopathic Physician. I think these are three of the most important to consider. I will close with the words of one of my mentors, Dr. Rick Kirschner, ND. (Go watch his incredible documentary, How Healthcare Became Sickcare: The True History of Medicine: https://talknatural.com/documentary.html) This is his "elevator speech" for Naturopathic Medicine, and I think it's beautiful:

"I am a doctor. I'm not an MD, a D.O., a DC or a PhD. I'm a Naturopathic Physician. I trained in a 4-year naturopathic medical school, where I learned the alternative to giving people petroleum derivatives and cutting off troublesome body parts; where I learned that an ounce of prevention really is worth a ton of bandaids, and that if you treat the cause of a problem you may be able to eliminate the problem, but if you only treat the symptoms, eventually they are likely to kill the patient. You could say that naturopathic doctors are the world's trained experts in natural medicine."

If any of these thoughts resonate with you…if you're looking to make positive changes in your health…you may want to consult with a Naturopathic Physician.

Sources

1. https://bit.ly/ras-rep
2. https://bit.ly/gall-dr
3. https://bit.ly/nd-scope
4. https://bit.ly/AMA-nutr
5. https://bit.ly/ND-nutr
6. https://bit.ly/CDC-Rx
7. https://bit.ly/Ther-Order

Dr. Alan Bradford, NMD *is a Naturopathic Medical Doctor who practices is Arizona. He is the co-author of* Please Bless the Refreshments: How to Really Nourish and Strengthen Your Body, *and the host of the popular podcast* Community Guidelines, *which features uncensored conversation about medical freedom, informed consent, and natural medicine.*

You can follow him on Twitter at:
@freethinking_dr

And read his Substack at:
https://doctorsnote.substack.com

Personal Success Story

by Jason Klietz
@Earbuds_music

In January 2011 I was given the biggest wake-up call. I had s blood clot that blocked the flow of blood to my brain and caused me to collapse and stop breathing. I was lucky to have first responders save my life. It took me months to learn the real value of having a second chance, so I set out to change my life. On the day this happened, I weighed 538 pounds and was very inactive. It took me nearly a decade to lose 100 pounds. My biggest issue was I didn't make the commitment to myself yet.

It wasn't till 2018 that I really started focusing on what it was going to take me to accomplish the task of getting healthy. 2020 when the world changed, I found reasons to stop working on myself rather than find ways around losing my ability to work out in the gym. In April 2022 I looked at photos of myself and couldn't lie to myself any longer about how far off track I had become and the effects of that were. I started working out again with the goal of becoming healthier. I was also learning that to become healthier, there are other changes that had to be made to achieve my goal of getting healthy. I shattered my world view and got to work rebuilding myself from the ground up.

I am just over 1 year into working on my goal of getting healthier in physical, mental, and financial health. This last year has been about character building as I have gone through an emergency surgery and a serious back injury. Without having the tools I have been building along the way, I wouldn't be where I am today. I am nearly healed from the back injury and once again got back up and on track to work on the next year of this journey. From April 2022 to April 2023 I went from 424 to 350. I am proud of my wins, also learned a lot from things that didn't go as planned. Overall, I have built a strong foundation to keep moving forward. Making this life commitment to myself is the best thing I have ever done.

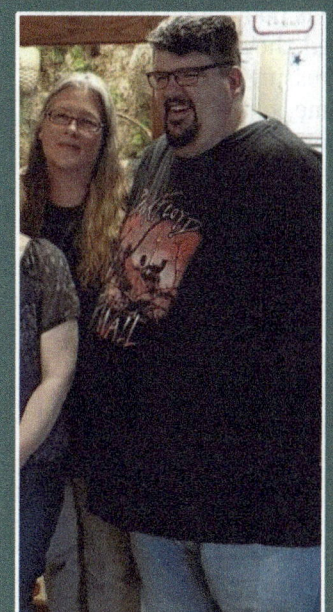

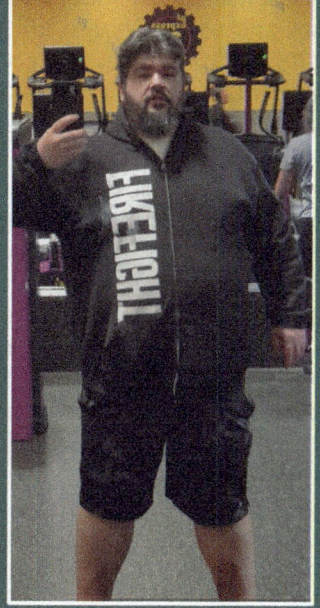

Disc Herniation: To Cut, or Not to Cut?

Andrew Lehn, MD

> "**I JUST** want this fixed", said an irate patient in a wheelchair coming in for an initial consultation.
>
> The patient had herniated a disc and was in severe pain. Knowing how excruciating nerve pain can be, I understood the patient's desire to stop the pain as soon as possible.

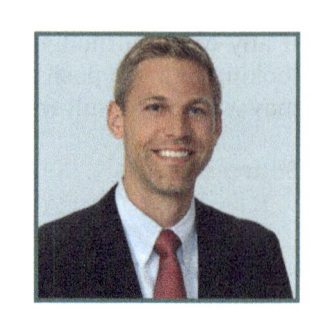

As 21st Century Americans, we are accustomed to easy fixes and clear-cut solutions to our problems. Unfortunately, the back is not a simple fix like other injuries. Once a disc or the spine is damaged, it truly never heals completely to how it was before the injury, even with surgical correction.

After the patient went on to talk about the work he had missed and his wife chimed in that something had to be done, I told him that 85-90% of patients with disc herniation do not end up requiring surgery. Since that is the case, it means that most people are able to get their pain under control and back to living normal lives without surgery!

The majority of pain from a disc injury is actually coming from spinal nerves. The spine carries the nerves to the entire body and when a disc herniates it can irritate surrounding nerves from inflammation and mechanical pressure from the disc pressing on the nerve itself. Unfortunately, a disc will never fully heal back to its original state. There is poor blood supply to discs and once they are injured they never return to their previous state. Discs pressing into the spinal space will get smaller with time, but they will never heal as strong as they were before the injury.

Even as the disc begins to heal, the nerve may continue to be painful. Nerve pain can be excruciating and frustratingly does not respond well to opioids. Opioids are great to treat acute pain from bone breaks, soft tissue injuries, and surgery, but often do little to help damaged nerves. In addition, once a nerve has been sensitized, it is more prone to irritation in the future. This explains why pain can persist or keep returning. So what is one to do?

The goal is to calm down the nerve pain. A nerve that is aggravated fires excessively. When an injury occurs, it is important for the nerve to send a signal to the brain to alert the body of damage. However, once the painful stimulus has occurred it is not necessary to keep feeling the nerve, especially when doing non-painful activities. The reason the nerve is firing excessively in pain is due to the way nerves send signals to the brain. Each nerve is receiving excitatory and inhibitory signals. Once a certain threshold of excitatory signals is achieved, a nerve impulse travels to the brain. A nerve that is injured or irritated is reaching the excitatory threshold with little to no stimulation. The injured person is feeling the nerve all the time, even with minimal stimulation.

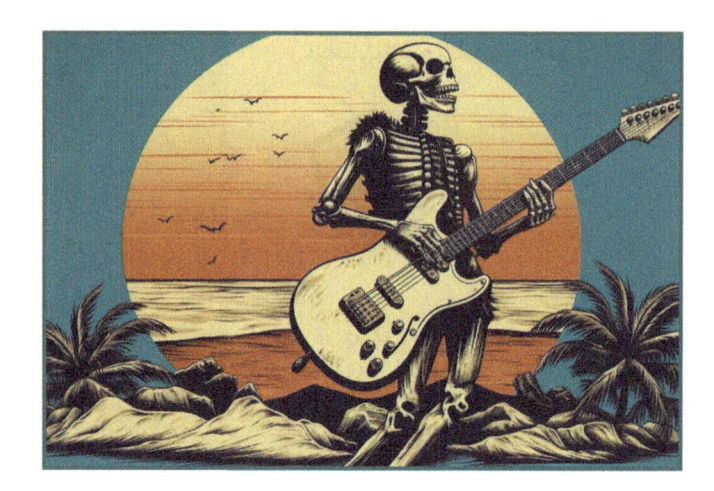

The goal of treatment is to raise the threshold that the nerve requires to fire and decrease the excitatory signals going to the nerve. There are several levels of treatment that are used to try to achieve this goal.

There are 4 levels of treatment:

Ultraconservative
These include non-invasive techniques such as Physical therapy (home exercises and professional guidance), Acupuncture, Massage, and over the counter medications such as Advil and Tylenol.

Conservative but non-invasive

There are several medications that help a nerve return to a less agitated state. These include steroids such as prednisone and medications that act on the nerve itself. These medications in two primary classes: SNRIs (a type of antidepressant but different from typical antidepressants like Lexapro and Prozac which are SSRIs) such as Duloxetine and Gabapentinoids such as Gabapentin and Lyrica. SNRIs work in the Central nervous system to help decrease pain signals reaching the brain, and Gabapentinoids work on the peripheral nerves to raise the threshold for the nerve to fire.

Conservative and Invasive

The most helpful injection for radiating leg pain is an epidural steroid injection. I like to refer to these injections as nerve injections rather than spine injections. The purpose of an epidural is to inject steroid as close to the affected nerve as possible in order to decrease the inflammation around the nerve and help stabilize the nerve itself. Steroids actually help decrease nerve hypersensitivity so it is more difficult for the nerve to fire in pain.

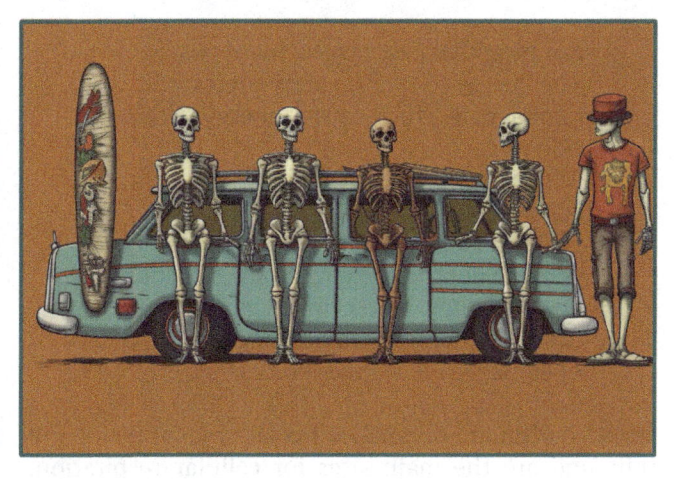

One of the most common questions surrounding steroid injections is "how long do they last?"

There are two ways to think about this question. On one hand, if the nerve is very irritated, it may not calm down with one injection. Occasionally, 2 or even 3 injections are needed to get a nerve that is aggravated to return to a normal resting state. On the other hand, they will last for as long as they do not get irritated again. Which means if there is a large disc herniation or significant stenosis, the nerve can keep getting irritated repeatedly.

Surgery

Surgery should only be undertaken to solve specific issues. It should never be used for generalized back pain. It should be considered if the pain worsens or keeps recurring despite repeated conservative efforts. However, if there is specific muscle weakness like a dropped foot, a surgical evaluation should be done expediently. Incontinence to bowel and bladder, numbness in the groin region, and sudden bilateral leg weakness is called cauda equina syndrome and is a surgical emergency. It indicates severe nerve compression and surgery is needed to decompress the nerve.

It is important to keep in mind that there are times a mechanical problem needs a mechanical solution. If a nerve is compressed to a large degree, it is possible that the pain will keep recurring until the compressing force is removed.

In conclusion, once the back is injured, it is essential to understand it will never heal to what it was before surgery. The damaged area will never regain full strength or resiliency. As a result, it is best to think about managing a spine rather than healing a spine. Fortunately, it is possible to manage a spine for very long periods without pain. Since most people have experienced back pain at some point in their lives, I believe everyone should be thinking about maintaining back health. Just as someone brushes their teeth to maintain oral health, I believe most people should be doing back exercises and controlling their weight to maintain back health.

Returning to my irate patient; he came back to the clinic after 2 Epidural injections and treatment with Gabapentin. He was back to work and just completed a cross-country flight with minimal pain. He actually apologized for his anger and was relieved that he had been able to avoid surgery. We discussed maintaining his exercise therapy, and I told him to stay in touch if the pain returned. That was several months ago, and he is still doing well!

Back pain can be debilitating, but there is a path to healing. Do not despair. Start the process and stick with it, and you can be living without pain sooner than you think.

Andrew Lehn, MD grew up playing sports every season and still looks to find avenues for competition and athletic endeavors. He was an avid Crossfitter and Spartan obstacle racer, and now enjoys water-skiing and local road races. He believes it is much easier to maintain strength and fitness than to let it go and try to find it again.

You can follow him on Twitter at:
@andrewlehn

ISSUE 2 SUMMER 2023

Mitochondria: The Missing Piece in Health Care

Anonymous

> **I AM** old enough to remember when there was no such thing as the internet. As far as healthcare was concerned, people had to trust their doctors, for better or worse. There was no googling symptoms, medications, or alternatives to overcome their illnesses.

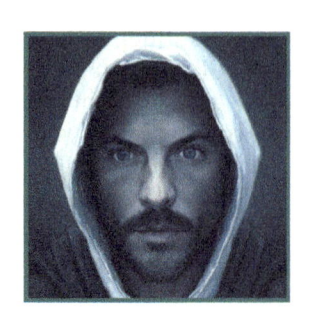

There were no blogs or podcasts people could subscribe to in order to gain different perspectives when it came to their healthcare.

Fast-forward to today. We certainly don't live in an information-less age. As a matter of fact, we have information overload. Depending on how you look at it, that could be a good thing or a bad thing. I say it depends. People often say, "If only I had more information, I'd be able to make better decisions!" That may or may not be true.

With so much information, people have a tendency to complicate things. I'm a simple man. I want simple answers and I've come to realize most people, at least with their health, think the same. Now, oftentimes there is not a simple answer. What I want to offer is low-hanging fruit solutions to common health issues. This, by no means, is me suggesting that we can eradicate all diseases. We all make choices we have to live with. Even if we're armed with the best information/recommendations in the world, we still have to go home and put the work in.

I'd like to offer you some advice to help optimize your health. None of this is medical advice, consult your physician before making any changes, and I wish you all the best.

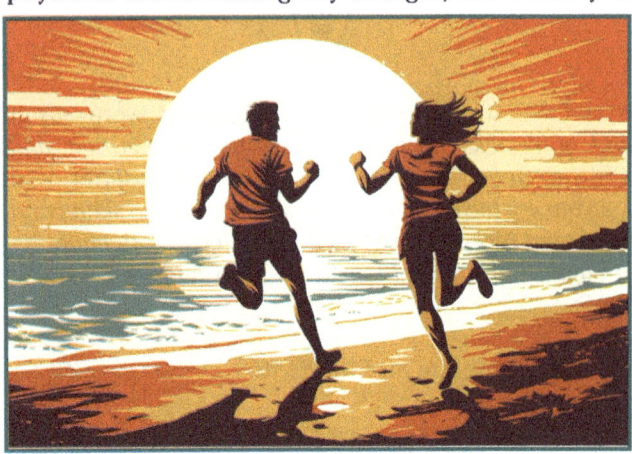

If you had a biology class, you've learned what mitochondria are. "Mitochondria are the powerhouse of the cell." Indeed, they are! Without getting too technical, let's recap:

- Running the body takes a lot of energy
- The energy to run the body comes from ATP (a molecule which carries energy within our cells)
- Energy from ATP drives every process in the body
- ATP production comes from mitochondria
- Outside of producing ATP, our mitochondria also produce water for our cells, aid in detoxification, stimulate apoptosis (death of damaged cells), and repair DNA

Mitochondria are organelles (small organs) inside our cells and are the main sites for cellular respiration. Cellular respiration is the process by which the human body extracts chemical energy from the food we eat. This, in turn, creates the necessary energy to carry out biological processes. The number of mitochondria varies. Some cells have no mitochondria, like red blood cells, and some have thousands, like liver and heart cells.

Mitochondria uniquely have their own DNA and can replicate without the cell dividing. Our mitochondria have little folds called cristae where most of the energy is manufactured. The outside membranes of our mitochondria are selective to what enters the inner membrane.

The moral of the story is, healthy mitochondria, healthy you.

It's important to have this basic understanding because, at our very foundation, at least in the physical sense, we are cells. Our organs, organ systems, muscle, bone, vessels are all made of their identifying cell type. Everything we eat, drink, inhale, and expose ourselves to will have a positive or negative effect on our cells. I always say, "Healthy cells, healthy us."

As we age, we lose mitochondria and the ones that remain may not function properly. Remember, our mitochondria are what produces the energy we need to live. Allowing for a healthy cellular environment gives us our best chance to be well.

We get our mitochondria from our maternal side. When we hear somebody say, "that person has good genes" (they're usually describing longevity), think of mitochondria. Think about this for a moment. Let's say your great-grandmother was a smoker, ate an awful diet, avoided the sun like the plague, and drank heavily. What is the quality of mitochondria your grandmother received? If your grandmother also had the same lifestyle as her mother, what is the quality of the mitochondria your mother received?

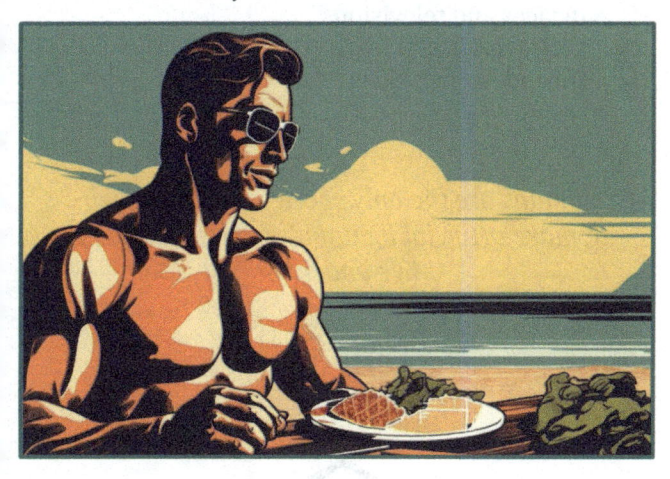

See what I'm getting at?

Now, that's not to say you can't break the cycle, nor do I believe somebody is doomed because of the choices of their grandmothers. What we must do is arm ourselves with the proper information and act on it. I once heard somebody say, "Some people are born 30 years old." They were referring to what I just described above.

How do we avoid cellular aging? We can't. Aging happens to all of us, some faster than others but that's why I'm writing this. I want to offer some examples of how we can optimize (I don't love that word) our mitochondria and age healthily. Some experts believe aging is a pathology. I'd say premature aging is a pathology.

Tip 1: You Are What You Eat
I'd say, more specifically, we are what we digest and assimilate, but you get the point. Nutrition is a hot topic and is very polarizing due to the diet camps and biases. Your body is the most magnificent, high-tech machine on the planet. You need to fuel it well. What diet is best for you is not for me to say. What I will say is consume real food including fish, grass-fed ruminants, fruit, eggs, and vegetables. Those should make up the majority of what you eat. Individual needs will vary.

Tip 2: Timing of Meals
At this point, almost everybody has heard of Intermittent Fasting or time-restricted feeding. A lot of people have had excellent results utilizing a smaller eating window, myself included. If you haven't heard of time-restricted eating, your eating window is much smaller than your fasting window. An example would be eating meals between noon and 6pm, then fasting until noon the following day. Many people have lost weight, improved their blood work, and were able to reduce/eliminate medication (only your doctor can do that, friends). Some research has shown that time-restricted feeding can enhance mediators to produce mitochondrial biogenesis and improve mitochondrial function and numbers.

Tip 3: Personal Care Products
Our skin is an organ. What you put on it matters. Try to be aware of the ingredients in things like soap, shampoo, conventional sunscreen, lotions, hair gel, etc. Constantly bathing our cells in chemicals that are harmful is a surefire way to damage mitochondria. This is usually a new one for a lot of people and can be overwhelming. The good news is there are many personal care products that are not harmful and aren't hard to find. Be patient, due your research, and you will figure it out.

Tip 4: Exercise
Of course! Any type of exercise is better than none at all, but we must move. It is well established that exercise can provide a powerful stimulus for mitochondrial biogenesis. The only disagreements seem to be what is *best* for mitochondrial biogenesis. A good approach would be a mix of cardiovascular (walking, jogging, biking, etc.) and resistance training.

Tip 5: Light Environment
If you were wondering if I was going to mention sleep, light environment and sleep go hand in hand. A quality light environment will help us sleep better. In my opinion, this last tip is the most important. If you had asked me 10 years ago what the most critical lifestyle intervention was, I would've said nutrition. Although nutrition is very important, I believe in the next decade, we'll continue to see more evidence that an optimal light environment might be the most

important lifestyle intervention.

I'll be honest. I went down a rabbit hole on this specific topic many years ago that I'm still deep in. It can be complicated, but I'm going to keep it simple and practical.

Let's talk melatonin. Melatonin is one of the most, if not the most, potent antioxidants known. Melatonin is produced within the mitochondria in response to sunlight and provides targeted protection of mitochondria from reactive oxygen species. Reactive oxygen species are highly reactive substances which contain oxygen radicals. Accordingly, melatonin is protective against a range of diseases including cancer, neurodegenerative diseases, cardiovascular disease, and diabetes.

Infrared radiation from the sun stimulates Cytochrome C Oxidase, which tells mitochondria to stimulate melatonin production. About 95% of the melatonin in the body is produced by mitochondria. The pineal gland produces the rest. The near infrared portion of natural sunlight stimulates an excess of antioxidants in each of our healthy cells and the cumulative effect is to enhance the body's ability to rapidly deal with changing conditions throughout the day.

To put it simply, intramitochondrial melatonin is a result of getting infrared radiation from natural sunlight.

Many people fear the sun. I'm here to tell you that you shouldn't. The easiest, most practical advice I can give you to fix your light environment is to have bright days and dark nights. Start the day with catching a sunrise. Spend 10–15 minutes getting morning sunlight and allow some sun to enter through your eyes. In other words, don't go outside with sunglasses. You don't have to stare at the sun. An added benefit of morning sunlight and skin exposure is that it builds what's called a "solar callus." Essentially, getting morning sunlight/skin exposure prepares and protects your skin for the higher UV rays during midday. A solar callus is what I like to call Nature's Sunscreen. You should also take a few short breaks throughout the day. Even if it's not sunny, the sun is still there, and the full light spectrum is present.

Depending on skin type, people can spend more or less time outside. I forgot to mention, I'm not condoning getting burnt. As a matter of fact, intermittent burning is dangerous. I don't recommend that, of course. The Fitzpatrick Skin Type Chart will give you a good idea of where you are and how to get safe sun exposure. The idea, however, that any sun exposure is dangerous is founded in quackery.

We also need to avoid artificial light, as much as we can, especially at night. Humans are not nocturnal. Our retinal cells (light sensitive cells of our eyes) have little metronomes that help regulate circadian rhythm (sleep/wake cycles). I mentioned earlier about the importance of exposing our eyes to sunlight. This is one reason why.

Blocking artificial light, especially blue light at night is a must. Artificial light at night suppresses melatonin production. What happens here is that light signal gets absorbed through our eyes and goes to a part of our brain called the Suprachiasmatic Nucleus (houses our circadian clock). This tricks our bodies into thinking it's daytime.

How to fix your light environment:

- Morning sun exposure
- Safe sun exposure throughout the day and watch the sunset if possible. Don't burn.
- Wear blue blocking glasses (400-550 nm) especially at night if you're looking at devices and televisions
- Sit by candles or a fire
- Incandescent bulbs

Humans are the only species bright enough to make artificial light and stupid enough to live under it.

Dr. Jack Kruse

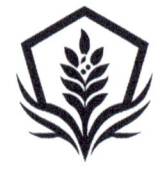

The Author *has been a direct primary care physician for 15 years and practicing BJJ for 11 years.*

You can follow him on Twitter at:
@ngdpc1

ISSUE 2 SUMMER 2023

How Medical Guidelines Work

BowTied Loon

> **IN** my last article for Renegade Health *(see Renegade Health Magazine Issue 1 Spring 2023)*, part of what I wrote was some tips on finding a physician who will *actually* help you optimize your health—making sure they're not going to just go through the usual guidelines and that they actually know (and practice) optimization.

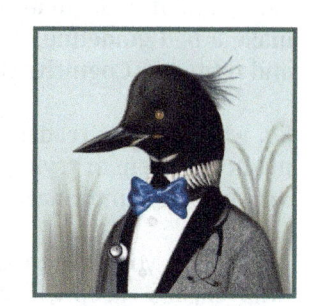

For this article, I thought I'd give a bit of insight into where the guidelines come from—while I'm not involved in this directly, I know people who are and have gotten to observe a bit.

First, let's take a look at who is involved in writing medical guidelines. I'm going to stereotype heavily here (because it works).

Mainly, they have to be academics. If you're not at [insert prestigious institution here], the chance that you get to be on a guidelines committee approaches zero. The problem here, to use a term by Nassim Taleb, is that they're all "IYI's"—"intellectual yet idiots"—which basically means that they usually have no real world experience. The example that Taleb uses is the business professor (probably at an Ivy League school) who has never run a business.

The issue with writing guidelines when your guideline writer is an IYI and doesn't have cutting-edge clinical experience is that they can't handle exceptions. I'd personally argue that the majority of medicine comprises exceptions. So in this case, when a question comes up that's not addressed by a randomized-controlled trial, they're clueless.

Example: try to find me guidelines on what to do for a patient with an LDL of 60 mg/dL who has severe atherosclerosis and continues to have cardiac events. Even better—ask the academic what they'd do in this situation, and then ask me.

Wait—a reply guy thinks he found a guidelines paper by a bunch of people who aren't academics? Wrong. This is actually an industry/pharma-funded guidelines article, where they often paid the authors and a ghostwriter. Good try though, reply guy.

The other thing that's hilarious about medical guidelines is that when they decide that something

---

Personal Success Story

by Ernie Stevens
@estevens0845

"You don't have a choice," were the words my trainer, IFBB pro, Rob Washington, would yell at me during my training session. Let me take you back in time and give you a glimpse into my fitness journey and where I am today. During my time at the San Antonio Police Academy in 1994, I was trying to gain some size and strength. I joined a local gym, Red's Gym, and became a regular gym rat very quickly. I was blessed to be in the presence of some amazing humans that helped me learn the gym culture. Within a few years, I purchased the gym and decided to give bodybuilding a try. In 2008, I competed in the NPC South Texas Classic as a novice lightweight competitor. I won 1st place in the first responder/military category, 2nd place in the novice category and won the show's overall best posing award. The bodybuilding lifestyle would continue to consume my love for the sport. In 2011, I competed again in the NPC South Texas Classic and won 1st place in the lightweight novice division and 3rd place in men's physique.

I eventually sold the gym and concentrated on building a mental health unit for the San Antonio Police Department. I felt the calling to help our community members that were diagnosed with mental health conditions. This was a huge undertaking, but the rewards of helping others has been incredible. In the fall of 2016, I was contacted by a filmmaker who wanted to film a documentary about the police department's mental health unit. After 3 years of filming, Ernie and Joe: Crisis Cops debuted at South by Southwest (SXSW) in Austin, TX, 2019 and won the festival's award for empathy in craft. The film, which can be seen on HBOMax, went on to win an Emmy and has been screened all over the United States.

(continued on the following page)

27

needs guidelines (easiest example here is Covid-19 vaccines, but there are others), they'll just make things up despite any data. Seriously: someone will be on a Zoom call and come up with a bunch of suggestions based on zero evidence, and everyone will nod and agree, and it ends up as a guideline. Worse: once they make a bad guideline, it's really hard to admit defeat and retract it. Cognitive dissonance is strong.

So, what can the reader, who is just trying to use the medical system or trying to help their family member, take from this information?

I'd say that you have to take ownership of your health. This means deeply studying up on any medical problems that you have—I advocate for doing your own research.

- Is health information confusing? Yes.
- Are you going to find conflicting and inaccurate information? Yes.
- Could you come to a completely incorrect conclusion? Yes.

But if you don't even try to learn about your medical problems, you're completely at the mercy of the system.

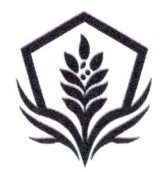

BowTied Loon M.D. *is interested in health and fitness performance, particularly regarding cardiovascular disease, longevity, and optimizing testosterone levels. His knowledge on these topics were gained by self-serving interest, since these things are not taught in medical school. BowTiedLoon is highly regarded in his real-life field, with a focus on diagnosing and managing rare, immune-mediated and genetic diseases. He actually has numerous publications in leading journals and could have pursued a university tenure, but instead chooses to run a successful medical practice and make money over a professor title.*

You can follow him on Twitter at:
@BowTiedLoon

And read his Substack at:
https://bowtiedloon.substack.com

(continued from the previous page)

In the winter of 2021 I decided to write a book about mental health. In March 2022, I released, Mental Health and De-Escalation: A Guide for Law Enforcement Professionals. The book went #1 bestseller on Amazon in the first week of release and can be ordered at ErnestStevens.com or directly from Amazon. The goal was to give first responders a better understanding on how to respond to mental health crisis calls.

But what about bodybuilding? I did compete a third time in 2018 in the NFF Alamo Showdown and won 2nd place open, and 2nd place Masters over 45. I have continued to train and will be competing in my final show in October 2023 in the NPC San Antonio Classic at the age of 52!

Bodybuilding has been my coping mechanism during my 28-year career in law enforcement. Lifting weights is a great way for me to work on releasing stress, and focus on something outside of work. First responders are placed in situations that cause psychological trauma and if good coping skills are not in place, your self-care will suffer. Diet, training, and support are the trifecta of a well-balanced life. Weight training will always be a way of life for me, and I hope it will be for you as well.

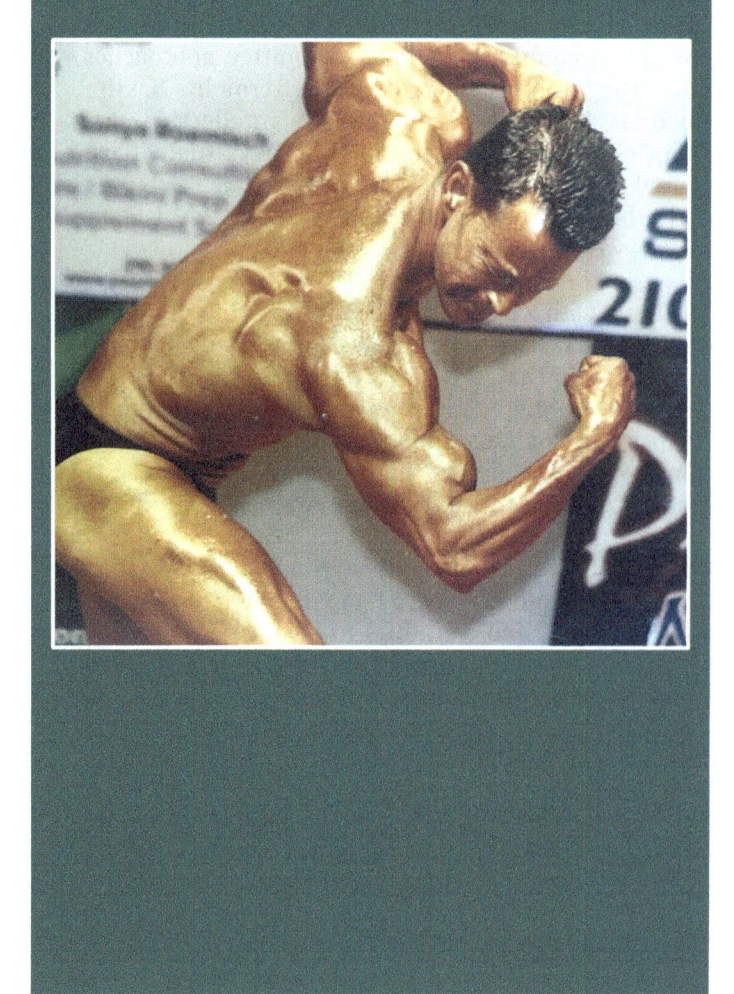

ISSUE 2   SUMMER 2023

Serum, Moisturizer, and How to Use Them

BowTied Fawn

> **WHILE** serums are used to deliver high concentrations of active ingredients in a water based formula, moisturizers are used to provide water and oil back into your skin barrier. Generally, serums are used to target specific skin concerns. For example, serums with vitamin C are used to improve your skin tone.

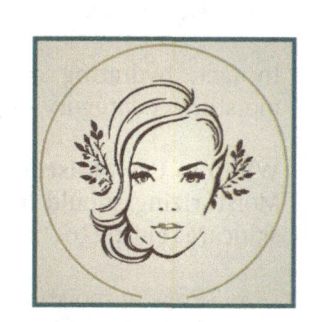

On the other hand, moisturizer can also be used to target specific skin concerns but are generally thicker formulas used to fight dryness and nourish your skin barrier. For example, moisturizers with retinol are used to provide anti aging benefits while also soothing dry skin.

That being said, there is some overlap between serums and moisturizers. For example, serums with hyaluronic acid are used to keep your skin hydrated, and some people consider these to be moisturizers too.

This article will explain everything you need to know about serums, moisturizers, the difference between them, and how to use them.

The Difference Between Serum and Moisturizer

While there is some overlap between serum and moisturizer, the big difference comes down to the inclusion of fats and active ingredients.

Serums are water based, while moisturizers often include emollients and oils to help deliver fatty acids back into your skin barrier. Further, serums tend to be lighter products while moisturizers may be heavier or greasier depending on the type of product you're looking at.

Most importantly, serums deliver highly concentrated amounts of active ingredients. For example, any popular vitamin c serum will have between 10-20% L-ascorbic acid. On the other hand, moisturizers have lower concentrations of active ingredients, if any.

This all being said, both serums and moisturizers are great steps to include in your daily skin care routine.

Serums

Serums are skincare products with high concentrations of active ingredients. Their exact purpose depends on your skin type and specific skin concerns.

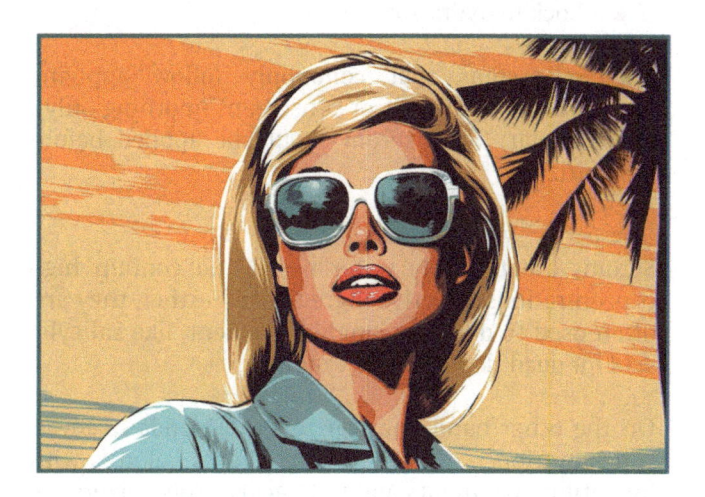

For example, individuals with oily skin or acne prone skin may benefit from a niacinamide or salicylic acid face serum as these ingredients have oil control properties.

Alternatively, individuals with dry skin may benefit from a serum with hyaluronic acid and aloe vera as these ingredients have great hydrating properties.

Other key ingredients in common serums include vitamin C serums to fade dark spots and retinol serums for collagen production.

When to Use Serum

You should use serum after cleansing your face and applying toner. Then, follow up with a moisturizer and potentially a facial oil depending on your skin type.

Moisturizers

Moisturizers are skincare products that provide fatty acids and hydration back into your skin. Using facial moisturizer is an essential part of a holistic skincare routine as it supports your protective barrier and fights skin irritation.

There are many types of moisturizers, including:

- Lotions
- Creams
- Gels
- Occlusives

In fact, hydrating serums may even fall into the moisturizer category, depending on who you ask.

When to Use Moisturizer
Moisturizing should be the last step in your evening skincare routine to:

- Prevent moisture loss
- Fight dry and flaky skin
- Lock in hydration

The only steps that commonly follow applying moisturizer are face oils or sunscreens (morning only). In particular, facial serum should be applied before moisturizer.

Serums vs. Moisturizers
Serums are typically water based and contain high concentrations of active ingredients. Further, they are often used to deliver a single ingredient, like salicylic acid for dead skin cells, for example.

On the other hand, moisturizers are blends of lower concentrations of active ingredients along with hydrating ingredients and fatty acids. Moisturizers are thicker and protect skin from cold air and harsh winds. That being said, both serum and moisturizer can be great additions to your skincare routine to improve your skin health.

Is Serum Moisturizer?
Certain serums toe the line of being considered moisturizer. For example, a hydrating serum with hyaluronic acid and panthenol might be moisturizing enough for people with oily skin. However, particularly for people with dry skin, serum is not a replacement for moisturizer.

Additionally, serums with high concentrations of harsh active ingredients should always be followed by a layer of moisturizer. For example, you should moisturize after using serums with:

- Vitamin C
- Retinol
- Glycolic acid
- Lactic acid

Among others. This is especially important for individuals with sensitive skin types.

How to Use Serum and Moisturizer
To use serum and moisturizer, follow this guide:

- Wash your face thoroughly
- Apply serum and gently rub in until absorbed
- Wait 1–2 minutes
- Apply moisturizer

And that's it!

You can layer serums if you wish, as long as it doesn't cause any irritation or other skin issues for you.

Should I use both serum and moisturizer?
You can use both serum and moisturizer if you would like to get specific benefits. For example, retinol face serum is used for anti aging while eye serum is used to get rid of dark circles.

Not everyone needs a serum, but most people will benefit from using a moisturizer.

Serum before or after moisturizer?
You should apply serum before moisturizer. Water based serum is lighter than any moisturizer. Therefore, you should apply it first. Remember, we always apply skincare from "thinnest to thickest" or "wateriest to oiliest".

Can I use serum instead of moisturizer?
Yes, you can use serum instead of moisturizer, depending on your skin type.

For people with oily skin or acne prone skin, a hydrating serum can be a substitute for moisturizer. However, people with dry skin will likely need to use moisturizer morning and night to prevent flaky skin and irritation.

Is it necessary to apply moisturizer after serum at night?
For people with dry skin, it is necessary to apply moisturizer after serum at night. Doing so provides continuous hydration to your skin and can soothe skin after serum ingredients like retinol.

However, people with oily skin may not be able to tolerate moisturizer without breaking out. In that case, just a hydrating serum is fine.

How long to wait between serum and moisturizer?
You should wait 1–2 minutes after applying your serum before applying moisturizer.

Can serum and face oil be used together?
Yes, serum and face oil can be used together.

Certain active ingredients in facial serums can cause dryness and irritation. By applying moisturizer and facial oil after applying serum, you can reduce these side effects and keep your skin healthy.

Serum or oil first?
You should apply serum before moisturizer and oil. Even if you skip moisturizer, serum should still come before oil.

What serums should I use at night?
The best serum for your nighttime skincare routine depends on your skin type and specific skin concerns:

- Mature skin: try out a retinol serum
- Dark spots: try a vitamin C serum
- Dry skin: try a hydrating serum
- Oily skin: try a niacinamide serum
- Blackheads: try chemical exfoliants, like a salicylic acid serum

Is it necessary to apply moisturizer after serum at night?
In most cases, you should apply moisturizer after serum at night. However, if you have particularly oily skin and are using a hydrating serum only, then you may be able to get away without using moisturizer after serum.

How long after serum to apply moisturizer?
You should wait 1-2 minutes before applying moisturizer after applying serum.

Summary: Serum or Moisturizer?
Both serum and moisturizer are great steps to include in your daily skincare routine, and there's no need to choose between them.

While serums deliver high concentrations of active ingredients and can help target specific skin concerns, moisturizers provide water and oil back into your stratum corneum.

Together, face serums and moisturizers work together to provide you with great, glowing skin. Just remember to apply face serum first and let it absorb before applying moisturizer.

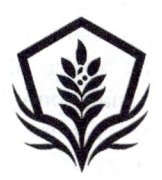

BowTied Fawn *is a pseudonymous author and private & commercial skincare consult. She writes Skincare Stacy's Stack through Substack, blogs through SkincareStacy.com, and is the co-founder of biöm, a personal care company.*

You can follow her on Twitter at:
@BowTiedFawn

And read her Substack at:
https://bowtiedfawn.substack.com

And shop her products at:
https://brushwithnobs.com

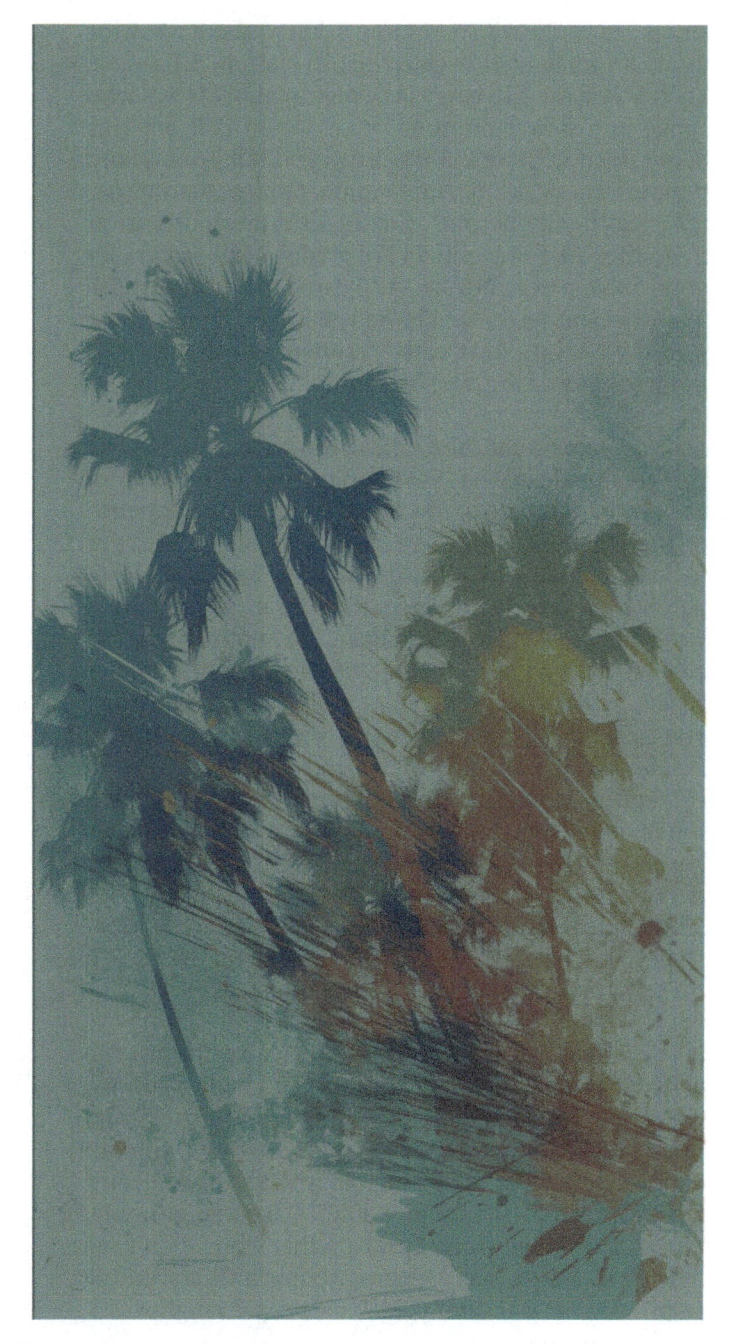

My Journey Through Drug Addiction

Alex Cherry

GROWING up we all hear the same lines from our parents and teachers. Things such as being respectful when someone is speaking, raising your hand if you'd like to say something, looking both ways before crossing the street, don't take candy from strangers, oh and the most important, DON'T DO DRUGS. I must have missed that lesson.

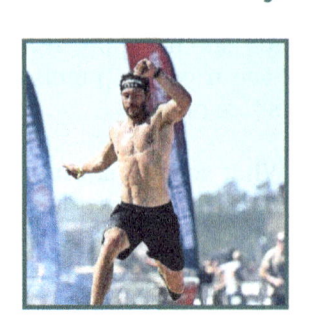

Drugs were always something I knew about growing up. I can remember back to health class in 3rd grade. My teacher, Mr. Pistner, a very nice man in his 50s who spoke in a slow monotone voice, would pull out this board filled with look-alike drugs and talk to us about their effects. "Cocaine, methamphetamine, marijuana, LSD, and finally heroin". I never paid much attention to it, after all, I was only in 3rd grade! What 3rd grader gives a damn about drugs. All I cared about was whose team I would be on for kickball that day at recess. No, growing up, I couldn't care less about drugs and cared more about making people laugh.

You see, I was what they call, a class clown. You know, that guy in class who makes an ass out of himself for the better good, or better laughter, or at the expense of the teacher's lesson. Yes, that was me. It was my identity inside and outside the school's walls. My parents had a messy divorce when I was 10 years old. I was the oldest of 4 siblings. My mother was an alcoholic who had a lot of untreated mental health issues, and it was ripping our family apart. I remember one time I came out of my room to go to the bathroom in the middle of the night and I heard a lot of commotion going on in my parent's room. I opened the door and saw my dad on top of my mom, slapping her in the face with a phone held up to his ear. I saw pills scattered all over the bed. I was too young to put 2 and 2 together, but I was told days later my mom tried to kill herself. My dad told me this on the way to the psych ward to visit her a few days later.

It was after that event that I started to turn into the class clown at school. Making people laugh made me feel good. The feelings I had at home were stress and pain. I looked around at my friends at school, who all had two parents at home. A mom who loved them, and a dad who protected them. I didn't have that at home. I had an alcoholic mother and a father who I didn't see much because he was spending so much time working to provide for our family. Making people laugh was a way out of it for me. It made me happy to make other people happy. I tell this part of the story because it's important. It's where my addiction was born. My addiction to running from my problems. My addiction covered up the pain in my life with something that made me feel good. It has been said before that addiction is a disease, and in my personal case, I don't believe that one bit. Addiction for me was hiding. Hiding from the negative thoughts and emotions I was feeling. Addiction was a warm blanket on a cold October evening.

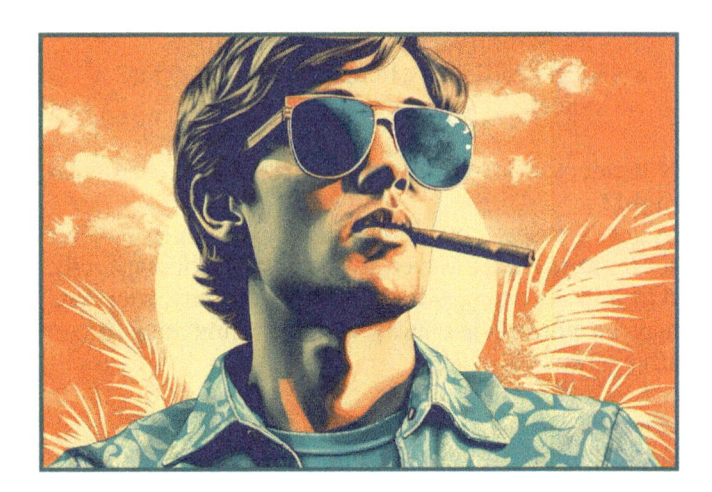

All through my high school life, I never messed with drugs besides booze and weed on the weekends. I never had any interest in them. Matter of fact, we kicked one of my friends out of our lunch table in 11th grade because we found out he was doing pills. My friends and I may have been the renegades of our grade, but we had some sense of morals. My vice in high school was still to make people laugh. It made me happy. People-pleasing is something that was born from the lack of love in my upbringing. I didn't have it at home, so I found it through laughter at school. Of course, this came at the expense of always being in trouble. I was a frequent flyer of detention, and later in high school, I would graduate to out-of-school suspensions. I didn't care though and viewed them as mini-vacations. I enjoyed them; my dad, not so much.

I was in trouble often growing up, and I didn't care. I had no regard for authority or anyone who felt like they could tell me what to do. I was on probation from 15-18 and then 20-21 and then again from 26-29. The state and I became quite close. All these cases centered around underage drinking and a DUI.

When I was 22 I got introduced to oxycodone, a prescription opiate painkiller. The feeling I got from that pill that night was euphoric. It made me feel a way that weed and booze never did, and the best part is that it took a quarter of the time. I started doing those pills once every few days, but it didn't take long for that window to dwindle down to every single day. One day the dealer went dry. The dealer had run out of pills, but in place of the pills, he had something else. Heroin. I told him I never touched the stuff and that I wasn't someone who did heroin. Well, that lasted 30 seconds because there was no other option. I took that first hit of heroin and my whole world lit up again. All the sickness I was feeling the past 8 hours went away.

This is the part of the story where it goes fast.

The heroin addiction grew by the hour. Each day my tolerance grew, which meant I had to do more drugs to achieve the same high I was accustomed to. It wasn't a problem for the first few months, but there came a time when I started running out of money. I thought about quitting, but that seemed impossible at the time. I couldn't go more than 2 hours without doing heroin so I had no faith in myself quitting for a whole day, let alone for good! But I needed money if I was going to keep doing it. I came up with a plan.

You see, I was a manager of a bar restaurant and had the codes for our computer system. My plan was this: Void customers' meal tickets after they paid and pocket the money. Horrible idea, but seemed like a bulletproof idea in my drug-induced haze. So that's what I did. Each day I had to steal more and more to buy what I needed. I was stealing over $300 a day from my job to support my drug habit.

Life was great in the spring of 2016. I had a good job, alright friends, and a 24/7 personal bank. That was until the Friday before Memorial Day. I got a call while I was getting ready for work, it was my boss.

"Alex, have you been deleting f**king tickets?".

I froze.

In 3 seconds the past 8 months flashed through my head and I felt my world slipping out of control. I didn't even try to deny it, I knew the jig was up. I admitted what I did and he fired me on the spot.

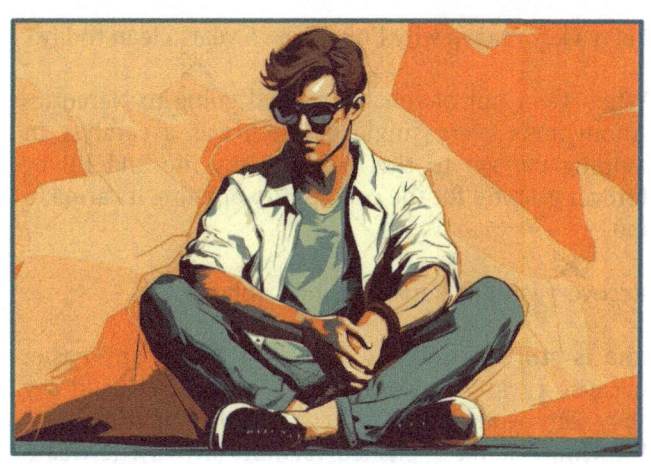

I sat on my floor after he hung up and cried harder than I ever have in my life. I figured my life was over, so I may as well go out with a bang. I grabbed the rest of my heroin and my gun and sat down at the kitchen table. I proceeded to snort every last drop of my heroin, and then pulled out my gun to finish off the job.

Before I could even load my gun, I heard my doorbell ring. It was a coworker I was close with who drove to my house to check on me after she heard the news.

She saved my life that day.

I would spiral out of control for the next 8 months before I went to jail for my crimes. In that 8 months, I stole thousands more from friends and family. Sold anything I could get my hands on and would have even ripped off my wonderful grandparents had they still been alive. I had no regard for anyone other than my addiction. I even admitted myself into the psych ward 3 times and stayed for a week each time because I had nowhere else to go and needed a place to stay.

Jail is where my new life began.

I was sentenced to 6 months in jail followed by 90 days in rehab. I had never been to jail before. I took the first time hard. You have a lot of time in jail so I did a ton of reflecting. Thinking about what my life would look like moving forward and how I could make amends for all the pain I caused the people around me. It wasn't until I got to rehab that my healing journey began.

My roommate, Todd, was a middle-aged alcoholic who had been in 10 previous rehabs. He told me he used to drink his girlfriend's perfume to get drunk. "Damn Alex, at least you weren't doing that!" I thought to myself. Todd was a key part in me gaining my confidence back in early recovery. The lessons he shared with me still sit with me to this day and have been a key reason why I'm almost 5 years clean today.

When I got out of rehab I started going to Narcotics Anonymous every single day. NA was a catalyst in helping me get to this point in my life and I'll be forever grateful for the community opening its arms to me.

Recovery isn't all sunshine and rainbows.

Life is still life and the hardships aren't any easier because I wasn't getting high every day. I would say they were worse because I could feel them. Whatever life threw at me I pushed forward anyway. It was a long journey to rebuild my life and there were thousands of times I wanted to quit. I went from being a confident man who everyone liked to be around, to the guy who stole a bunch of money from his job and a drug addict.

But through hard work and determination, I pushed through the storms and came out on the other side. I could never have imagined the life I have today. It's still surreal to think about. I feel blessed to have been given this second chance in life.

I've helped dozens of addicts over the past 4 years see this new way of living as well. An unfortunate fact is most of the addicts I worked with in NA relapsed weeks and months into recovery. They couldn't wrap their mind around the fact that life wouldn't always be this way—that if they showed up every single day and put in the work that their life would change as well.

It's a grind, but like anything in life worth having you must put the reps in daily to achieve your desired result. Recovery has taught me more about myself than I ever learned in the first 25 years of my life. It calloused my mind in the sense that little things in life don't bother me anymore. I mean come on, I was a heroin addict for 3 years, went to the psych ward 3 times, went through heroin withdrawal DOZENS of times, went to jail for 7 months, and had to rebuild my life from scratch. With a past like that, it's hard for anything worse to happen to me.

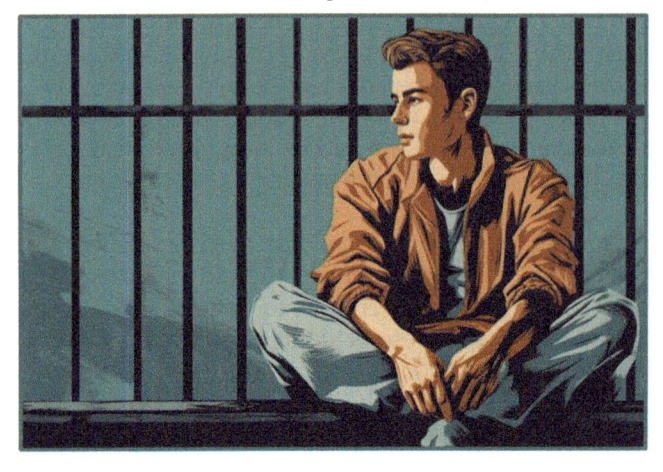

It comes down to perspective and awareness.

For the first 2 years of recovery, I had little confidence in myself. I thought everyone saw what I saw in myself. What did I see you ask? I felon ex-drug addict who had to prove himself. I wasn't wrong, I did have a lot to prove to my community and more importantly, myself.

I put my head down and pushed through all the bad times these past 4 years that got me to the exact spot I'm in now. Anything meaningful in life worth having is going to take a lot of work, and recovery from drug addiction is no different. I would venture to say it's going to take even more work in that case. Put the work in, and you'll reap the rewards.

The problem with that is, like most things in life, people would rather try to achieve a goal but at the first sign of adversity, they crumble. They clench their fists and yell at the sky, "why me!?!" Then they quit. They have a fixed mindset. They can't fathom that their life can change with the proper motivation and hard work. I call that group the victims. The people who always have a story about why something didn't go according to plan. The excuse-makers. The negative Nancy. The people you want to avoid in your life when you're embarking on something meaningful and amazing because they will try to put their dark clouds over your progress.

I had a few of those victims try and latch onto me at the start of my journey. I had enough wit to tell them to buzz off. Negativity and complaining solve nothing. It does nothing more than waste precious energy that you could use to propel yourself forward to amazing successes.

If you tell my story and leave the drug part out of it then it's a story about a man who went through some hardships and decided enough is enough. He put his head down and got to work and constructed a whole new life for himself despite the mountains of adversity in his path.

It's a story about grit and determination.

Most people have a story like that and can relate to it. Even the people who say "I never had to work that hard." Maybe you haven't, but I'm sure you have a story from your life when you had to work hard to achieve something. Think about one of those times in your life. Did the task feel impossible? Did you somehow manage to come out on the other side successful? Do you remember how you felt when you achieved what you wanted to?

Think of that time. Never lose sight of that memory. Pull it out when times are tough and you need the motivation to push forward. I use my personal story as motivation daily. It's my personal gas station when life seems impossible. It's what helps me gain perspective on my life. If I said, "I can't" to my grandma, she would quickly fire back, "you mean you won't!" What are the things in your life that you *can't* do? The things in your life that you think are out of reach and not possible for yourself. Replace the *can't* in your life with "**I will…**"

See where that takes you in life.

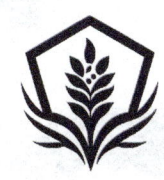

Alex Cherry *had a $400 dollar-a-day heroin addiction 6 years ago. Through the grace of god, his family, an amazing support group, holistic health, and a 7-month stint in jail, he can tell you how he became 6 years heroin free and never felt more blessed to be alive today.*

You can follow him on Twitter at:
@alexwcherry

And see his website at:
https://sustainfitness.co/

Signs and Symptoms of Addiction

Narconon: https://www.narcononus.org/resources

Get Help Now: CALL **(877) 805-9430**

Physical Signs and Symptoms of Drug Use and Addiction:
- Bloodshot eyes
- Pupils larger or smaller than normal
- Changes in appetite or sleep patterns
- Deteriorating physical appearance or grooming
- Unexplained weight gain or loss
- Unusual smells on breath, body, or clothing
- Impaired coordination or tremors
- Changes in behavior
- Lack of energy or unusual bursts of energy

Physical Harm Resulting from Addiction:
- Heart and lung damage
- Cancer
- Hepatitis and HIV
- Liver damage
- Stroke
- Tooth damage and loss
- Impaired immune system
- Kidney damage or failure
- Brain damage

Changes in Quality of Life:
- Declining performance at work or school
- Deteriorating care of children, spouse or home
- Legal situations
- Traffic accidents or multiple tickets or loss of one's license
- Arrests for drugs, disorderly conduct or assaults
- Loss of job, business or home

Behavioral or Mental Problems:
- Erratic mood and behavior
- Risk-taking, such as reckless driving or promiscuity
- Being anxious, depressed, paranoid or fearful
- Suffering delusions or hallucinations
- Appearing foggy or spaced out
- Borrowing money repeatedly
- Poor memory
- Unexplained changes in friends or hobbies

Narconon Arrowhead. Signs and Symptoms of Addiction. https://www.narcononus.org/signs-drug-addiction/. March 30, 2022

ISSUE 2 SUMMER 2023

Why Man Needs Emotion

The Trauma Guy

THERE has been the impression that strong males do strong male things without emotions. While it's true that we can function to a limited extent with limited mastery of emotions, if one wants a higher level of masculine mastery one must dive into the emotional world.

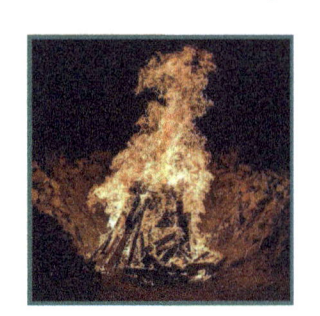

Ok Trauma Guy, that sounds extreme, emotions are feminine, you sound crazy! Crazy maybe, counterintuitive, yes, which is why we will start off with the martial arts. In higher levels of martial arts, there are two aspects of "Stealing Time" that will make a warrior nearly invincible. Sensing intent and hitting your opponent before they move both require emotional competence (emotional openness and training). I was bummed no one told me the secrets held in a rare Japanese Swordsmanship book. Years later, I found my selected martial art expected these skills in their black belt tests, a method of bad guy exclusion.

An example is the masculine attribute of security. After a wonderful dinner, I was walking my date home and got the sense of "something wrong." Some would call "spidey sense" and after a quick scan I identified 40 yards behind me what appeared to be a tweaking drug user. After securing my date's safety, I went to investigate. It was a tweaker, but also didn't add up, so I decided he also needed help. I did a weapons scan and called 911, assisting in a safe transition to the cops. What was supposed to be "speed" for an aspiring college student turned into a bad trip.

My prior idea of security was to constantly scan for threats, see my exits, and have my back to the wall. Now, all that I desired from martial arts came from emotional clarity and without effort. Masculine areas of protection, security, providing, and intimacy are now enhanced.

How is this done with emotions? With a little discussion of the effects of trauma injuries, you'll soon understand a big piece of the puzzle. First, we all carry trauma. It can be inherited, received in utero, and we get a lot in childhood. As a result, we have triggers, parts of our body shut down, we stop feeling sensations and emotions because they hurt and are unpleasant. One can't throw a hard punch if the body shuts down the arm. We need to remove the blockages and remove the body/mind distortions created by the trauma years ago.

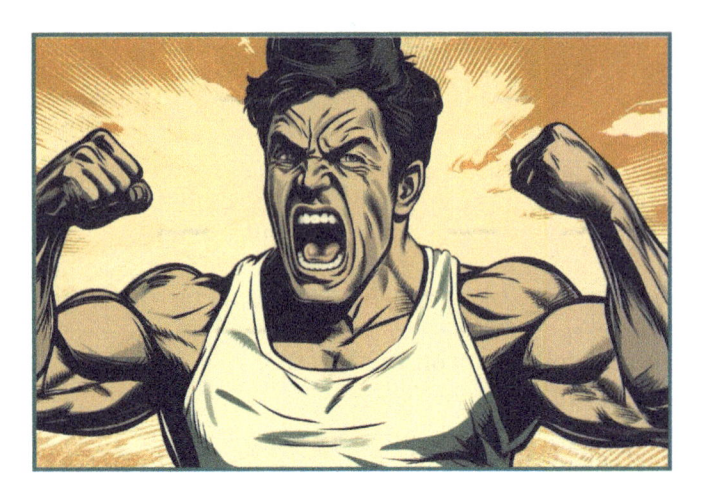

Here is where the magic of allowing emotions comes in! Time to hunt down the memories of our past and allow them to resolve. We open up to trauma release. For men, I suggest no-talk body workers. There is no need to talk, or explain, or understand. One can get crazy sensations, emotions, and memories to develop. Some are strong enough to watch them go by like clouds on a summer's day. Talk therapy can be a little fluffy and doesn't have the immediate results possible with somatic body work. For my clients, the goal is to assist them enough to where it's their natural process, no dependencies! If you are going to therapy and happy with the relationship, I would also augment it with a somatic body worker for faster results.

The results: emotional triggers disappear, along with the events that inspired them. Triggers that drop your IQ and cause a chemical avalanche in the body, shutting down healthy systems, go away. Imagine a good chunk of time without them and the productivity you will gain. Body / mind distortions go away, tensions disappear, health emerges.

Blocked body signals will reappear, which increases body wisdom. You will have more empathy and less judgment.

With continued work, all of your masculine attributes are enhanced. You provide security, protection, and emotional maturity. Your significant other will be attracted to the stronger version of you, and achieve levels of intimacy previously unimagined.

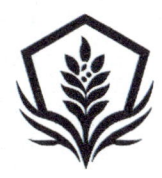

The Trauma Guy *has been practicing and receiving trauma release for 20 years. His knowledge comes from analyzing the results of trauma release and reading many esoteric and self-help books. His "story" of trauma release is functional, in that it "works", and may not be complete.*

You can follow him on Twitter at:
@TraumaInformd

Personal Success Story

by Stacy Pendleton
@spendleton01

I've been on my fitness journey for 7 years now. I lost over 80 pounds. I wanted to become healthy for myself, my girls and grandson.

When I started my journey, I was lifting a little to tone and was a runner. I ran a few 5k's, a 25k and finally ended that chapter with a marathon.

I decided to really get into bodybuilding after seeing I was transforming my body. I then set a new goal to becoming a bikini competitor. I found my true passion and my new chapter of my fitness journey.

It's been an amazing journey so far and I feel the best I have in my life. I just want to be an inspiration to others and let them know it's never too late to start! I started at the age of 45.

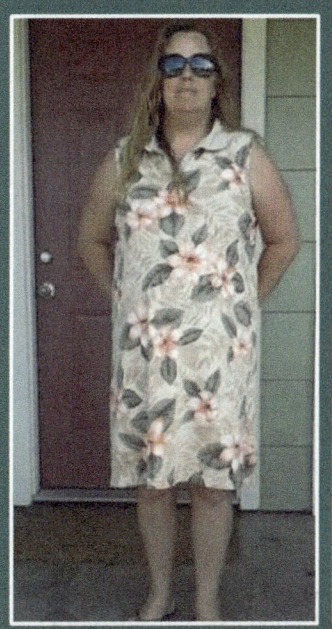

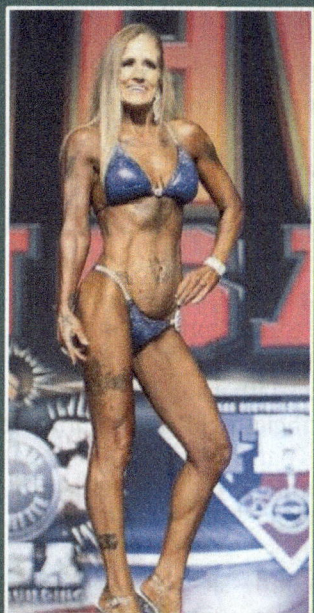

ISSUE 2 — SUMMER 2023

Your Daily Meditation Practice

BowTied Fighter

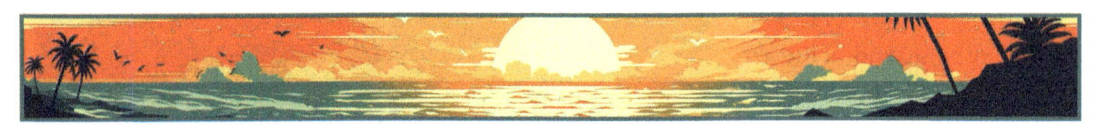

> **READ** this part out loud three times:
>
> After I read this article, I will sit down and meditate.

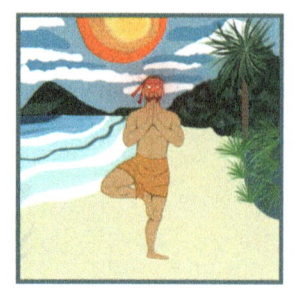

Maybe you have never meditated before. You are aware of the practice, familiar to an extent of what it is "meant" to do, maybe you even have some general idea of how it is done.

Right now we are going to go from absolute base level of the mountain and get you to climb a couple of hundred feet up the mountain.

After that, it's simply a matter of you deciding and continuing to climb.

Starting Your Practice
First, find a room or a space that you're sure will be as quiet as possible. When first starting out, it's best to practice in a space that is quiet. Minimize potential distractions, after all, meditation is rooted in being here in the present moment!

PRO-TIP: Esoteric blood memories tell me to avoid artificial light during practice. Try to keep your space as "natural" as possible! Taking this concept a step further, if the weather is nice go do your daily practice outside.

Second, sit down on the floor in a cross-legged position. Put left leg over right leg. Straighten your back. Sit down with dignity and take pride in how you sit! (Have some self-respect!)

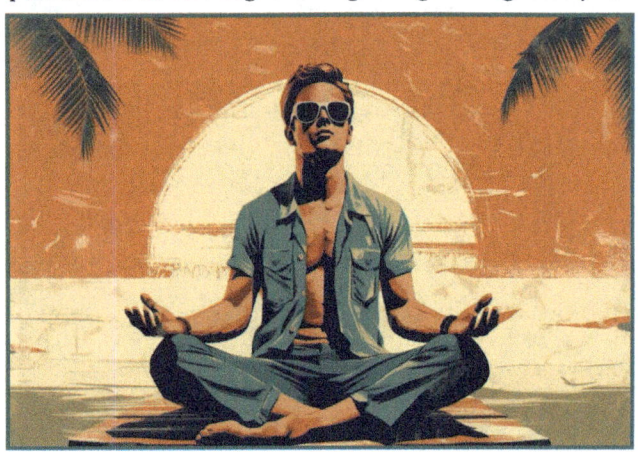

⇒ Maintain an upright, but not rigid posture. Keep your back straight, imagine a piece of string that goes from slightly above your head, down through the top of your head, down into your spine and pelvis area. Now, gently pull that string upward without making the line excessively taut. That feeling of being upright is what you are going for.

⇒ Relax your shoulders downward, unclench your jaw and let your tongue gently rest at the top of the roof of your mouth. Facilitate good breathing!

⇒ Place your hands on your knees or fold them in your lap. Whichever you choose, leave your hands there for the duration of time. Be resolute! Pick something and stick with it. You decide halfway through you want to put your hands in a different position? Do that next time you practice.

Mobility Issues
Not being able to sit cross-legged on the floor is A FLIMSY excuse to not meditate! Own a bed? Oh... Nice! You can meditate! Lay in bed, relax yourself downward and follow the practice the same way anyone sitting would do. If you can sit regularly then you can sit down in any chair that allows you to sit upright! It is even okay for the chair to have a back so you can have some support in sitting upright.

Third, set a timer on your phone for 10:30. Your practice is ten minutes long, the thirty seconds is a warm-up. In these thirty seconds, settle into your pose. Establish it. Close your eyes, draw neck circles to the left, then to the right. Roll a few forward circles with your shoulders, then a few backwards. While doing the above, start to become aware of your breath.

38

⇒ SHORTEN, DON'T SKIP! Five minutes is better than no minutes of practice, three minutes is better than no minutes. Remember the seeds? This is how you water them. SHOW UP!

Fourth, breathe. Simple. Just breathe. With your eyes closed, start breathing in through your nose, out through your nose. Just breathe naturally and comfortably in and out of your nose. There are levels to this—we are at level one.

Bring your awareness to your breath. This is where we start to meditate. Place your attention (your focus) gently onto your breathing. Feel the inhale come into your nostrils, feel the exhalation go out of your nostrils. Notice the physical sensation that happens when breathing. Make a mental note of the spot where you feel air come in & go out. Your awareness on your breath is placed at that contact point.

Be aware of the location where your breath goes when you inhale it into your body. Humans carry a lot of stress in their bodies. We spend a lot of time hunched over looking at phones or at our desks. This affects our posture, which affects our breathing. The change in posture makes it harder for us to breathe into our belly. What we end up doing is chest breathing.

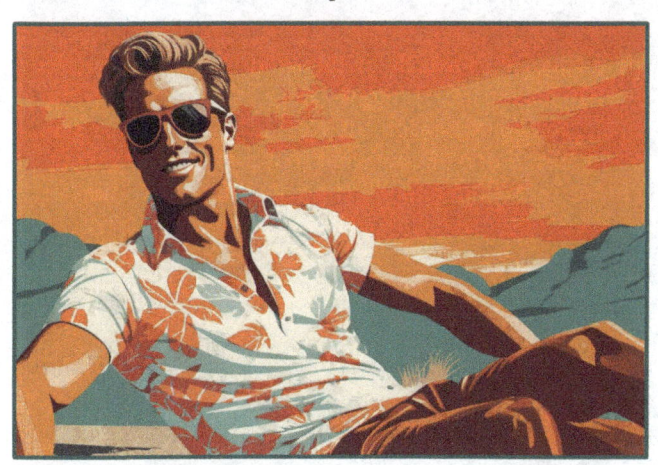

Simple Science: Air entering our lungs stimulates various lobes in the lungs. In these lobes we have nerves that control our Sympathetic Nervous System and our Parasympathetic Nervous System. The two parts of the nervous system serve very different purposes. The top portions of our lungs have nerves associated with the Sympathetic Nervous System. The lower portions of our lungs have nerves associated with the Parasympathetic Nervous System. When you breathe into your CHEST the Sympathetic Nervous System is stimulated. When you breathe into your belly and engage your diaphragm the Parasympathetic Nervous System is stimulated.

The Sympathetic Nervous System sends signals to our organs that stimulate them & prepare them for action. Short, shallow, hasty breathes into our chest (like how you breathe when you are under a ton of stress or when you are frightened) switch on the sympathetic nerves. The body redirects blood flow from non-vital organs to vital for survival organs. Your heart rate increases, adrenaline is released into the bloodstream, blood vessels constrict, mind focuses, etc. The Sympathetic Nervous System is heavily affiliated with a term I am sure you are familiar with, your "Fight or Flight Response." It's called this for a reason. When it's active your brain and body is in survival mode. Needless to say, excessive and continuous chest breathing will keep you in a high stress state!

The Parasympathetic Nervous System signals to your body to enter a state of restoration and relaxation. When the Parasympathetic Nervous System is active signals are sent to your stomach to digest. Signals are sent to the brain to pump hormones like serotonin and oxytocin into the bloodstream.

These are feel good hormones. The Parasympathetic Nervous System influences salivation, tear duct function, it even influences the loosening of the bowels to prepare for excretion of waste. Also, respectfully here people, it stimulates the genitals to prepare humans for sex. When you breathe into your belly and you engage your diaphragm, the diaphragm inflating stimulates those lower lobes of your lungs which activates your Parasympathetic Nervous System. You may have heard of this system by the name of the "Feed and Breed System".

Fifth, Rinse & Repeat (R&R) for the duration of your practice. All you need to do right now, is be aware of your breath. Feel it as it comes in, feel it as it goes out. Be here with It.

⇒ If you notice that your awareness has left your breath, simply note it in your mind and bring your awareness back to your breathing. Do this every time you find yourself noticing you are no longer present with your breath. You may need to repeat this process hundreds of times in your practice, or only a few. Either way, your ability to be aware of your breathing while meditating is something that is built with continuous practice.

What about when thoughts come into my mind?
For now, just bring yourself back to your breath. Thoughts are water drops in a bucket; intense for a moment but ripple out fast. Worry about them later.

BANG BANG. You just meditated, my brotha (or sista)!

I beg of you, keep it simple. The simpler your practice, the easier it is to remain consistent. Meditation is a long haul type of investment. You sow seeds today, they grow down the line. They have to be sown in order to grow though my gangsters!

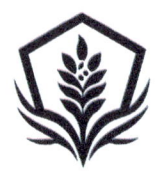

BowTied Fighter *helps people breathe better, relax their mind, live presently and have more energy.*

You can follow him on Twitter at:
@BowTiedFighter

And read his Substack at:
https://bowtiedfighter.substack.com

Personal Success Story

by BowTiedDaddy
@BowTiedDaddy

Sitting in the office chair, my fourth child sleeping in the stroller, I watched intently as the neurologist scoured over the genetic panel notes that just came back.

"Excuse me sir, I have never heard of this before, please wait while I go to my office and read up a bit." Stammered the doctor.

I immediately knew something was wrong. When she was born, I could tell there was something wrong, I just couldn't put my finger on it, but when he looked at the gene panel, his face validated all my negative thoughts.

"Sir, your daughter has something called PACS1, also known as Schuurs-Hoeijmaker's Syndrome. It is a genetic condition that causes moderate, life-long cognitive and physical developmental delays." Said the doctor in a shaky, choked up voice.

He might as well have been speaking Chinese. I had no idea what he meant. Thoughts were racing through my head but for some reason all I could think of was this question. "Doc, I don't know what that means, can you put it in terms I can understand? The only thing I can think of is Down's Syndrome. Is it like Down's Syndrome, Doc?

I will never, in my entire life forget what he said in response. "You WISH she had Down's Syndrome." He spoke, as he stared at the floor.

I'm sure he didn't mean to put it so bluntly. He was a nice enough guy. I'm sure he was just as stunned as I was, but those six words broke my soul. From there, I began my downward spiral.

I had already put on a few pounds during the pregnancy. Maybe 15 pounds of "sympathy weight", but after hearing the diagnosis, that was nothing compared to what would follow.

I started drinking every night.

I remember going to Costco and buying a handle of bourbon every other day. The nightly drinking, zero exercise, and eating like shit continued for about year. A year-long downward spiral of self-destruction and depression had caused me to gain 80 lbs and lose any resemblance I had of my old self.

(continues on page 45)

Zookeeping ADHD

Jordan Taylor

IS Attention Deficit Hyperactivity Disorder (ADHD) real? Ask that question and watch people's heads explode. But it's an important question because all mental health disorders are created by a small group of psychologists. They identify symptoms, guess at a cause, write it down in a book and – poof – it's real! Let the diagnoses begin.

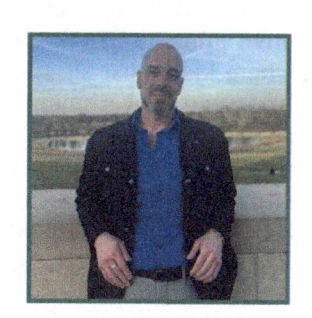

In 1968, they created ADHD. Since then, over six million children have been told they have the disorder.

But is it even real? It's an important question. Psychologists have been responsible for all sorts of mental health related horrors in the past. Doctors used to perform lobotomies (the surgical removal of brain areas). They thought they were doing the right thing. It was science. But lobotomies are no longer performed today. They stopped being real.

So, how should we approach the reality of ADHD? It depends on your perspective. If you look at the disorder from two different viewpoints, you'll get two different answers.

First, let's consider the mainstream perspective. Experts in the psycho-pharmaceutical industry tell us ADHD is a brain problem. According to professionals, people with the disorder have a chemical imbalance in their brain. These broken brains result in *abnormal behavior*, including poor impulse control, an inability to focus, disorganization, and restlessness. In other words, the location of the problem is inside the individual. That's why ADHD patients are treated with pills. Inject amphetamine into the brain and behavior will change.

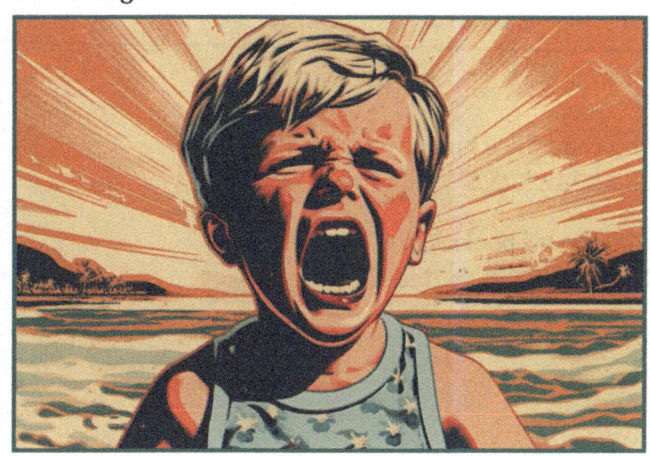

Now, consider a second perspective, the perspective of a zookeeper. Does that sound crazy? Good. Stay with me. You're about to learn how zookeepers are better at treating mental disorders than psychologists.

Over the last one-hundred years, zookeeping has evolved. In the early 20th century, most animals were kept in barren, concrete cubes with barely enough room to move. In these conditions, zookeepers noticed that many animals developed strange behaviors not seen in the wild. The odd behaviors included self-harm, excessive pacing, head-weaving, and over-grooming. Animal experts call these behaviors stereotypes.

Zookeepers knew they needed to solve the stereotype problem. What did they do? Did they decide the animals had a chemical imbalance? Did they reach for pills? No. Zookeepers took a different perspective. Instead of labeling stereotypes as abnormal behavior, they defined them as *behavior indicative of an abnormal environment*. In other words, the location of the problem is outside the animal. This is a crucial difference. There's nothing wrong with the animals. The environment they live in is wrong.

With the correct perspective, zookeepers started a movement called environmental enrichment. The St. Louis Zoo explains: "In the wild, animals must find food, defend territories, escape predators, and build homes. In zoos, the majority of animals' needs are provided by the keepers, so other methods of physical and mental stimulation must be provided to encourage natural behaviors." Today, zoos are now different. Enclosures include gyms, nets, and swings. Animals work for food in stimulating ways like freeing a piece of fruit from a block of ice. And members of the same species are often housed together to enhance socialization.

So, what happened to the abnormal behaviors once

the environment changed? You guessed it. They went away. No pills necessary. No invoice from a psychologist.

Now, let's use the zookeeper perspective to look at ADHD. Are people operating in an abnormal environment? Think about a classroom full of desks where kids must sit still all day and be yelled at by a low-wage government employee. Think about a cubicle farm with fluorescent lighting and never-ending spreadsheets. Think about a factory floor with poor ventilation and ceaseless noise. Think about a cramped apartment with one window and stacks of useless consumer goods.

You're in the human zoo.

Now, back to the question at hand. Is ADHD real? It depends. If you think it's abnormal behavior that comes from a broken brain, then I say no. But if you think ADHD symptoms are behavior indicative of an abnormal environment, then I say yes – because that perspective is empowering. It's hard to change broken brains, but it's easy to fix the environment.

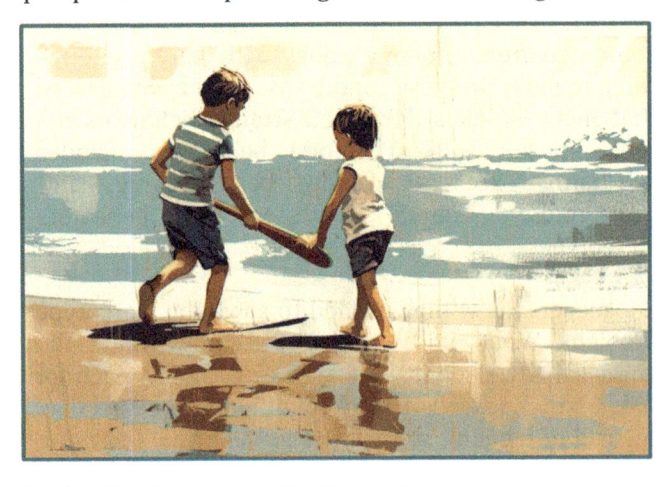

If you, or someone you know has ADHD symptoms, try the following before turning to pharmaceuticals:

⇒ Reduce clutter in your environment. Most of us have way more stuff than we need. In addition to creating a psychological burden, an excessive amount of stuff takes time and effort to clean, organize, and manage. A dose of minimalism can do wonders for attention.

⇒ Find or create opportunities for physical activity. Is there a gym nearby? Join it. Do the kids have open spaces to play? Find the nearest park. Sitting all day? Get a standing desk. Own some dumbbells, a yoga mat, exercise bands. Leave them where you can see them. Take the stairs.

⇒ Bring nature into your environment. Humans evolved in the natural world. Living things, plants and animals, soothe our psychology. Populate your home and workplace with greenery and low maintenance pets.

⇒ Manage your social groups. People are part of your environment. Who do you let into your life? Avoid too much interaction with energy thieves. Use distance and boundaries to minimize exhausting relationships. Of course, you may not socialize at all. Fix this. You need time with friends. Humans, even introverts, are social creatures.

⇒ See food as part of your environment. There is no mind-body split, so whatever goes into your mouth influences your psychology. Are you underfed? Stock your home with an abundance of food. Make it easy to eat. Overfed? Don't allow junk to enter your home, school, or workplace. The problem will fix itself.

Some of these suggestions will resonate. Some won't. The point is to start viewing ADHD with a zookeeper's perspective. What's happening on the outside? Which external levers can you pull to change behavior indicative of an abnormal environment? Start thinking this way and you'll avoid the pills and therapist bills. There is a better way. After all, the environment is within your power to control. Your brain is not.

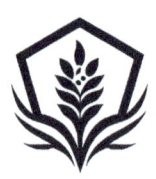

Jordan Taylor *is a U.S. Navy Master Training Specialist with a master's degree in teaching from Missouri Baptist University. He was diagnosed with ADHD as a kid and put on a daily dose of amphetamine. He got off ADHD medication as an adult and never looked back. He is the author of several books including Total Attention Magic, a guide that teaches parents how to help their ADHD kids without dangerous pills.*

You can follow him on Twitter at:
@attentionfixed

And get his books at:
https://jordantaylor.gumroad.com

Is Our Medical System Beyond Hope?

Brian Lenzkes

> AS a physician practicing medicine within the system for over 20 years, I have come to realize that our system is broken. When I first joined a practice, I showed up with my freshly pressed white coat and stethoscope, ready to save the world. I chose a career in medicine so that I could help those in need as well as provide financial security for my family.

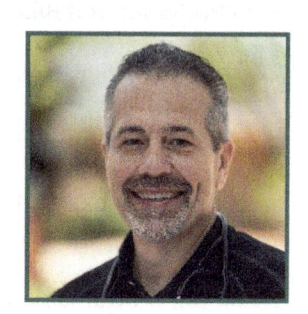

Over time, I realized that the more time I spent with individual patients, the less my income and the longer other patients would have to wait to be seen. Every year I noticed that I was becoming a cog in the wheel. I was rewarded more for efficiency and coding skills than I was for spending time with patients and getting to the root cause of their illnesses.

We have increasingly pitted physicians against patients in recent years. Physicians are overwhelmed by a dysfunctional system and a never ending supply of patients with chronic illnesses. The patient visits have been cut to 9–12 minutes on average, and doctors are spending more time in front of computers and following guidelines for reimbursement. Patients are also feeling like numbers as they're rushed through an impersonal factory system. It's apparent that modern medicine is on the wrong path for healing and the system is failing both healthcare workers and their patients. We have traded the genuine human connection for algorithms and guidelines. We have lost the ability to use critical thinking and personalized medical care for the person in front of us. Fortunately, I left that system 3 years ago in order to focus on patient care without the burdens of insurance oversight.

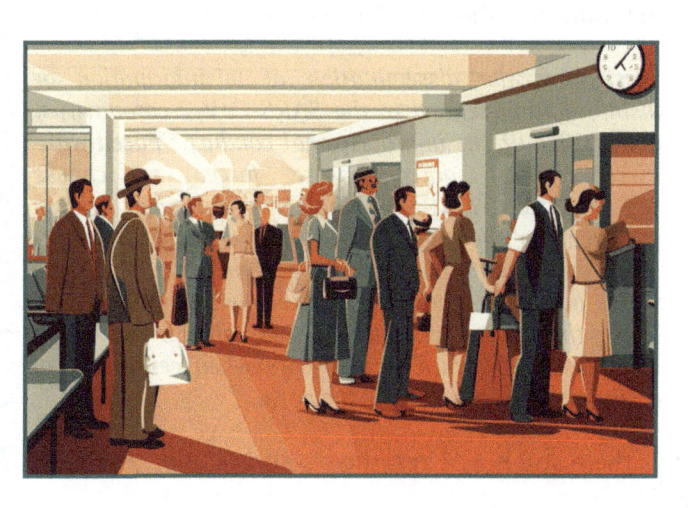

To make this case, I would like to share the story of one of my new patients. Let's call her *Janet*. She came to me hopeless. She was told by her previous physician that she had type 2 diabetes which is a chronic, progressive, and irreversible disease. She was on multiple doses of insulin daily and her sugars were out of control at over 450 on most days despite increasing doses of insulin. She also has a history of coronary artery disease with stents placed and multiple medications for this. She carries diagnoses of hypertension, obesity, hyperlipidemia, osteogenesis imperfecta (a disease characterized by brittle bones and multiple fractures), and an anxiety disorder.

When I asked her why she consulted with me as a Direct Primary Care (DPC), she said, "You're my last hope. I've done everything the doctors told me to do but I'm gaining weight and my sugars are worse than ever. If this doesn't work I'm going back to cookies and donuts." She was given the same advice over and over despite the fact that nothing was improving. In recent months she had gained over 25 pounds as her insulin doses escalated. She was on a vegetarian high grain diet because she was told this is heart healthy. She was told not to exercise because of the risk of fracturing more bones. In short, she was on a disaster course toward kidney failure, dialysis, blindness, amputation, and cardiac bypass surgery. As a result, she was suffering from anxiety and hopelessness. She was lost and the system was failing her.

Janet listened to her doctors and followed their directions perfectly, yet she was getting worse daily. Nothing that she tried worked and she was constantly hungry and fatigued. No matter how much insulin she injected, her sugars worsened and her hope faded. Her doctors told her that she was "non-compliant" and that she needed to work harder at improving her health. They could not fathom that their professional advice was poor.

Her previous physician did not have the time to discuss the importance of metabolic health and lifestyle in a 9-minute appointment. We spent 1 hour discussing the importance of metabolic health. This can be summed up briefly with 5 points that I learned from Professor Ben Bikman (PhD BYU):

1. Watch your stress, don't work yourself to death
2. Get adequate sleep
3. Eat real food
4. Don't smoke or drink to excess
5. Exercise regularly

These are 5 attainable changes that we can all make but are rarely discussed in modern medical clinics staffed by overwhelmed physicians. Doctors just don't have enough time to address these issues, and most are struggling with these same issues in their own lives. They don't have enough time to open this can of worms and therefore prescribe more drugs in order to feel like they're making a difference.

I speak from experience as I was working 16-hour days filled with chaos and stress. I was typically waking up at 4:30 AM in order to get a brief workout in and drive 35 minutes to the office to properly care for my panel of 2200 patients. If I left late, my commute time would double. I was constantly sleep-deprived (which is a badge of honor among doctors) and felt stressed if I "wasted time" doing nothing... Like spending time with friends and family. I was on a treadmill going too fast. I could manage it in the short term but I knew it was unsustainable for the next 20 years. I watched the physicians around me struggle with severe burnout and apathy. We were all drowning but were too busy to help each other to safety.

Janet is now filled with hope and remains determined. She is exercising most days with a trainer specialized in treating patients with mobility issues. Her sugars have improved dramatically while cutting her insulin usage by 75%. How can this be? It's critical to understand the importance of metabolic health and insulin resistance. It's the same concept as alcohol abuse. We initially get the desired effect with one or two drinks but with time we develop tolerance. If a patient presents to a physician's office stating they're drinking 12 beers a day and can't get drunk, what should they do? The standard approach is to continue increasing the alcohol until they get the desired effect. The patient is resistant to the pleasurable effects of alcohol so they need more and more to get the same effect. A wise physician would recommend cutting back on alcohol intake over the next several weeks. Then the patient wouldn't need 12 drinks to get the effect; one would do the job. The same is true of insulin resistance. If we continue injecting more and more insulin, the cells of the body become more resistant to insulin.

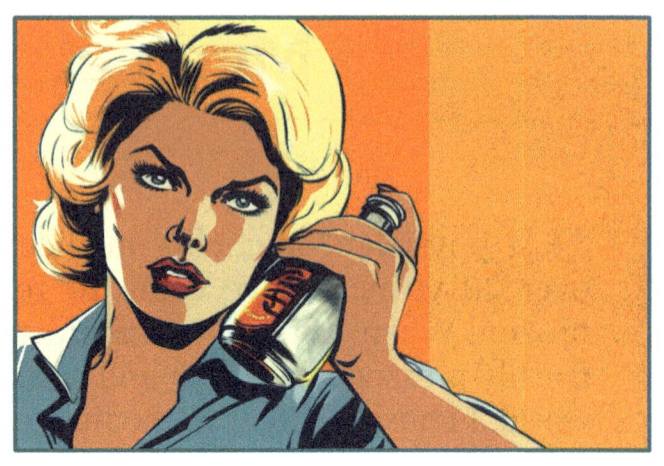

Insulin is the driving force for fat and sugar to enter the cells. It also inhibits fat breakdown, thus explaining why Janet had recently gained 25 lbs. Those 5 things that Dr. Bikman was talking about all improve insulin sensitivity, thus lowering sugar levels and improving health.

We are all facing life challenges. We're surrounded by processed foods and immense life stress. We're sleep-deprived and overwhelmed. We don't have time to exercise or pursue hobbies that bring us peace. We live in divided communities and lost our connections with each other over the past several years. We've been masked and isolated, which is the perfect breeding ground for loneliness, depression, and substance abuse. Many were abandoned by their family physicians because of personal health choices during the pandemic. It's commonly known that physicians were losing financial bonuses if their patients didn't follow standardized guidelines. Administrators place immense pressure on physicians to stay in line and follow rules. Thinking outside the current standard of care was considered dangerous and physicians were threatened with losing their licenses if they questioned current guidelines based on their clinical experience. The most devastating has been legislation in California called AB 2098 which:

"designates the dissemination of misinformation or disinformation related to the SARS-CoV-2 coronavirus, or "COVID-19," as unprofessional conduct." Faced with these threats, doctors were forced to choose self-protection rather than honestly assessing the risk vs.benefit for the patient in front of them. As a result, many outstanding physicians are fleeing to surrounding states in order to practice medicine without the fear of losing their livelihood. Medicine has always evolved by open discussion until recent years when censorship of opposing views has become the norm."

Is there still hope? Yes, there's always hope. We have

to become partners in health. Physicians must once again focus on the best option for the patient in front of them. We must once again focus on patient autonomy and informed consent which are the foundation of medical ethics. We have to act on behalf of our patients and stand in the gap for them, despite massive pressure from above. We have to focus on the root causes of illness and spend time in education. We must surround ourselves with like-minded professionals dedicated to outstanding patient care. Sometimes the best medicine is a smile and human connection. We must get back to our roots in order to save the medical system and ourselves.

Brian Lenzkes *is an internal medicine doctor based in San Diego who has focused much of his attention on clinical nutrition. He owned his own medical practice with a group of physicians from 2004-2020 until transitioning into an independent membership-based practice, San Diego Metabolic Health & Direct Primary Care (formerly LowCarbMD San Diego). A professional speaker in the health and wellness sphere, Dr. Lenzkes also hosts the Life's Best Medicine podcast and co-hosts the popular LowCarbMD podcast, which have a total of more than 5.3 million downloads.*

You can follow him on Twitter at:
@BrianLenzkes

And see his website at:
https://arizonametabolichealth.com

(continued from page 40)

I would show up to work, red-faced, sweaty, and breathing heavy. No-one said a word to me about it. All my "friends" were too scared to approach me about my weight because they felt bad for me.

"He's got a special needs kid, leave him alone." They would say under their breath.

I didn't need that, I needed someone to tell me to get my shit together...but no one would.

I had to do it myself.

One day it hit me.

As I looked at my daughter, I remember thinking to myself, "What the fuck am I doing!?" "Do I want to drink myself to death and not be alive to take care of my daughter?"

"Do I want her sisters to have to care for her because I was weak and couldn't get my life together!?"

It was at that moment, I decided to make a change.

I started working out, eating clean, and most importantly quit drinking. I took my life back, one day at a time. Using my daughter, and the rest of my family as motivation, I lost 70 pounds in just under a year.

There is more to be done.

The work is never over.

I will continue to show up every day for myself and my family.

But at least I have my life back.

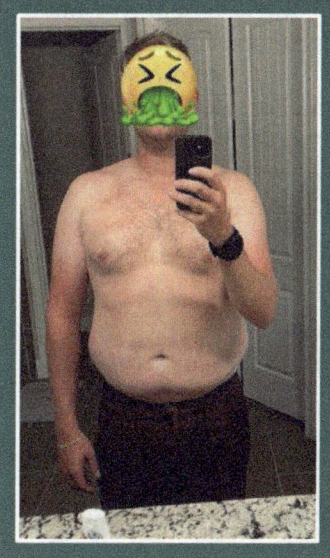

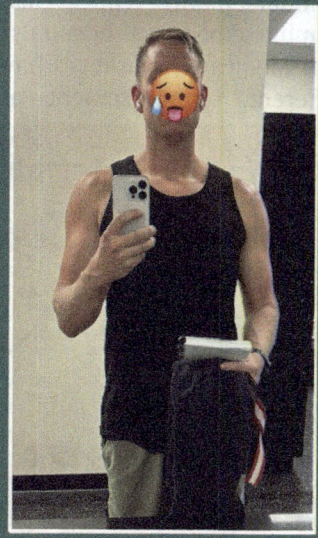

ISSUE 2   SUMMER 2023

Understanding Your Cost of Care

BowTied CEO

FOR many Americans, getting hit with a large medical bill can be shocking. You see these large amounts and the amount that you are responsible for fluctuates depending on your insurance, the procedure you had, or if you've reached your deductible. Let's try to make sense of this black box that is the cost of healthcare.

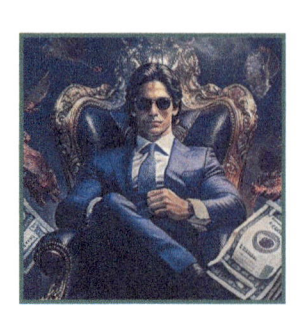

It All Starts with Medicare

Believe it or not, all medical bills start with Medicare. You may be asking, "How is my medical bill affected by Medicare, when I don't have Medicare as my insurance?" The Center for Medicare Services (CMS) determines what the reimbursement amount should be for both Hospital and Physician services each time you have a hospital stay, procedure performed, or you go to see your primary care physician. This amount is then paid by Medicare, or an administrative insurance company, to the hospital or physician who performed the service.

The Medicare reimbursement amounts are determined by a segment of the AMA made up of physicians and industry appointed officials known as the RVS Update Committee (RUC). Each year they update these rates based on certain changes to medical guidelines, laws, increased costs etc.

For private insurance, either through your employer or an open exchange, Medicaid, Medicare Advantage, VA, or Tricare, the insurance company uses the Medicare reimbursement rates as the baseline for reimbursement to hospitals and physicians. These non-Medicare insurances have the right to negotiate different reimbursement amounts depending on specific factors. These negotiated amounts could be more or less than what is set by Medicare. Generally speaking, non government insurance reimburses more than government insurance.

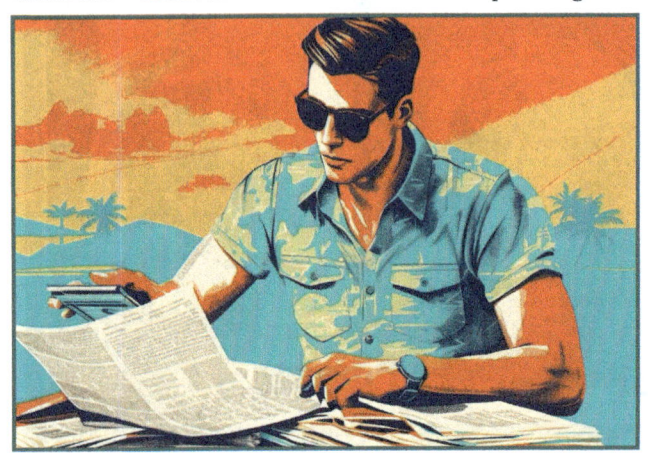

Once these amounts are determined, depending on what type of insurance you have, you will pay a portion for the services that were completed.

How Does Medicare Determine Reimbursement Amounts?

Medical billing is broken down by Hospital and Physician services due in large part to physicians owning private practices and having a physician's services agreement with a hospital to perform procedures in their facilities. Medicare, recognizing that still exists, determines reimbursement the same way. This is also a reason why, oftentimes, you will receive two separate bills. One for the Hospital facilities and one for the physician's time.

The Physician reimbursement amount determined by Medicare is based on a fee for service model, where each service the physician performs has a CPT (Current Procedural Terminology) code assigned to it, along with a reimbursement amount. These amounts vary slightly depending on geographic location and inpatient or outpatient setting, but are based on the average salary of physicians and the degree of difficulty for the procedure. These are updated annually by a government appointed committee.

Hospital billing is not as cut and dry. Each year, hospitals need to submit a Medicare Cost Report that breaks down all the operational expenses for providing care to patients on a per-case basis for the prior year. The expenses are broken out between labor and non labor, and become the basis as to how Medicare will reimburse the hospital.

The non labor portion includes things like medical supplies, pharmaceuticals, rent etc. The labor portion consists of all the salaries of the employees of the hospital, ranging from a nurse to the CEO. It includes any employee who works directly with patients and administrative staff.

Once the labor and non labor base payments are established, Medicare then applies adjustment factors for geographic location, inflation, and weights based on the complexity of the case, to determine what the reimbursement amount should be.

Medical Bills Explained

Medical bills can generally be broken down into four areas:

- Total Charges—What the hospital/physician bill to you or insurance
- Total Adjustments—The contractual reduction between total charges and total payments
- Total Payments—amount the insurance or employer pay to the hospital or physician
- Balance/Patient Responsibility—the amount you owe

The total charges are the aggregation of all the services that were completed for your particular case. This is what is billed to you or your insurance. Generally speaking, what the hospital or physician charges is arbitrary, unless you do not have insurance.

Most insurances have a negotiated rate with most hospitals and physicians that override any charge amount that the hospital or physician bill.

As an example, let's assume the negotiated rate with your insurance for a general consultation with your primary care physician is $100. If the physician charges $200, they will still only receive $100. If you do not have insurance, you would have to pay $200.

In very few cases, there are insurances that do negotiate to pay as a percentage of total billed or they can also negotiate a "lesser of" stipulation. An example of a "lesser of" scenario, based on the example above, would be where your insurance negotiates a rate of $250 for a consultation with your primary care physician and the physician charges $200. Your insurance would pay $200, the lesser of $200 or $250.

Aside from the uncommon instance where these scenarios occur, hospitals and physicians also have to be cognizant of price competition adherence with the FTC. The FTC will investigate any major price changes if they are notified by the public about egregious price differences or if the hospital/physicians group has a large market share.

The total adjustments are simply the difference between the total charge and the total payments. This is what the hospital is contractually obligated not to collect.

The total payments, as stated in the previous sections, are what the insurance is contractually obligated to the hospital for services rendered. This is important because it can affect how much the patient's balance is. As you reach your deductible or if you have very good insurance coverage, you will pay less of a balance each time you have services completed within that plan year.

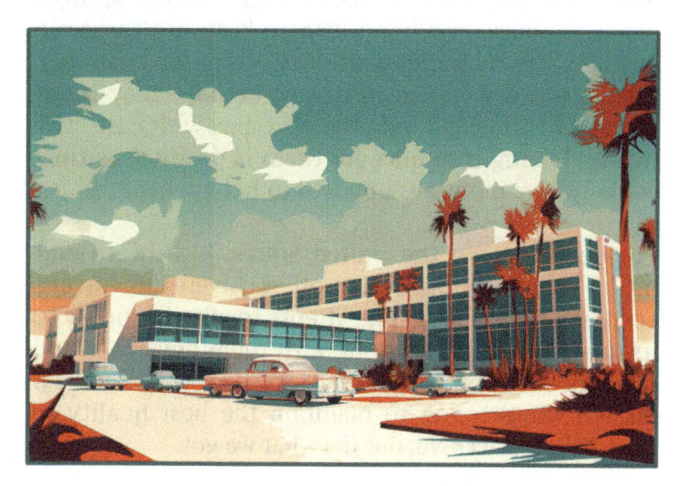

How Do Hospitals and Physicians Co-Exist with Insurance?

Healthcare and insurance actually have competing priorities. Hospitals and physicians make money as they perform more services. Insurance companies make money from people paying premiums, but do not use their health insurance. On the one side, healthcare profits when you are sick and on the other, insurance profits when you are healthy. How is this sustainable?

The first reason is that medical services are expensive. Would you get that knee operation that costs $20,000 if you did not have insurance? Probably not. If your total out-of-pocket max is $15,000, you just saved $5,000. The savings is even more if you add on other services along with that knee surgery, like pain medication, physical therapy, and post surgery nursing care.

Why Does Healthcare Have To Be So Expensive?

Healthcare workers are paid well in the United States. Physicians and nurses in the U.S. make more than most other countries for the same position. Insurance allows them to get paid. If private insurance did not exist in the U.S. and it adopted universal healthcare, we would have a bigger shortage of healthcare workers and we would end up like the U.K. with quality issues and physician labor strikes. Insurance and healthcare feed off of one another.

The second reason is that accidents happen all the time. Even if you are considered healthy, you don't want to take on a potential large financial burden. If you want to run that risk, feel free. You never know what tomorrow holds. Do you want to have a mountain of debt because you did not want to pay annual premiums?

The third reason is that Americans are sick and they are not getting better. The United States is the overwhelming leader in obesity, and we aren't slowing down. Obesity related diseases like diabetes, high blood pressure, and heart disease keep healthcare in business. Obese patients are cash cows for hospitals. They also need health insurance because they reach their deductible and out of pocket max with ease. The ROI on having insurance for them is positive, as they actually save money as opposed to not having it.

To summarize, in the United States, healthcare and health insurance need each other. Given the current economics of healthcare, patients require hospitals to fix something that is wrong with them physically and insurance steps in to alleviate some of that financial burden while trying to maintain the best quality of care. Is it perfect? No, but it's what we got.

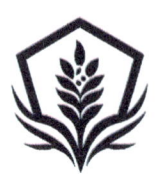

BowTied CEO is the Corporate Chad of the back office. Decision maker for the decision makers. Insight into the inner workings of the C Suite.

You can follow him on Twitter at:
@BowTiedChadCEO

And read his Substack at:
https://bowtiedchadceo.substack.com

Personal Success Story

by Daphne

As an immigrant from the Philippines living in Maui, I've learned the importance of a healthy diet and lifestyle. My family and I have been following this lifestyle for at least 15 years. We go to bed early, wake up early, and eat mostly home-cooked meals. Even when we're on vacation, we make sure to maintain our healthy habits.

When my kids were young and I was a stay-at-home Mom, we would go to the library every Tuesday afternoon and I would borrow recipe books and cooking magazines to learn how to make delicious and beautiful meals. My husband taught me the basics of cooking. He now says, it was the best investment of his time.

It's not always easy, but it's worth the effort. Since 2004, I've been preparing meals for my family, making sure we have a healthy breakfast, a packed lunch, and a nutritious dinner every day.

Through reading, I've come to understand the connection between diet and health, and I want to age gracefully. I'm not obsessed with avoiding certain foods, but I am fastidious about how the foods we eat affect our well-being. We've made healthy eating a way of life, prioritizing foods that are the best and densest source of nutrition.

To make healthy eating convenient, I stock up on foods we like that are mostly healthy and simple to prepare. We always have food with us to avoid being tempted by unhealthy options when we're out. We mainly buy locally sourced, pasture-raised, organic, or wild foods, even though they're more expensive. It's worth the cost because these foods are more nutrient-dense, keeping us fuller for longer and giving us more energy.

By prioritizing our health through healthy eating and lifestyle habits, my family and I have been able to maintain a happy, healthy life.

ISSUE 2

SUMMER 2023

The Bitcoin Cure

Anonymous

I HAVE always dreamt of becoming a physician. I feel grateful to have fulfilled that vision. At the same time, I'm disappointed by how different the reality of the job is from my expectations. I imagined my career would involve healing people, seeing their illnesses go away, and transforming their lives.

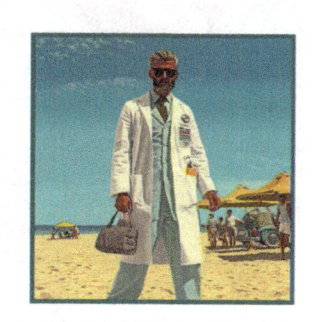

Instead, I work in a system that aspires to only "manage" disease and hide symptoms with toxic medications or invasive surgery as patients continue their overall downward health spiral.

I work as a Hospitalist, which is an Internal Medicine physician for hospitalized patients. While my viewpoint is biased in that I deal with the sickest people in the community. Americans are remarkably unhealthy. Despite the US spending nearly twice on healthcare as other high income countries, it still ranks among the lowest on various health measures.[1]

The decline in healthcare quality despite rising costs is often blamed on free market economics. There is a general belief that selling healthcare for profit is only good at making greedy pockets bigger. But people have always been greedy. Why are we only now feeling its effects on healthcare? Having spent more than a decade in the healthcare system, I have concluded that the problem is not in people's love of money, but rather in the money itself. This paper will attempt to elucidate that connection. We start off by showing how the US healthcare system is not a free market enterprise, we will then discuss how this separation from the market is maintained by our current fiat dollar backed monetary system. Finally, we conclude by explaining how Bitcoin, an alternative to fiat money and modern central banking, can fix many of the problems in modern healthcare.

The US is often touted as an exemplification of free market failure in healthcare. This could not be further from the truth. Due to restrictions on the supply and demand of services, US healthcare has turned into a public/private hybrid benefiting a few but not its patients. It combines state mandates of seemingly private insurance companies, as well as restrictions on the licensing and number of providers in a system highly susceptible to regulatory capture by pharmaceutical companies.

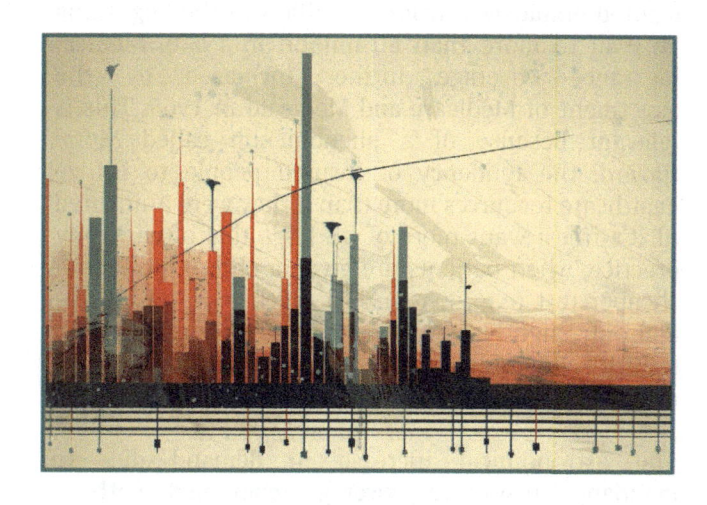

On the supply side, in 1903 the American Medical Association (AMA) was formed. Its main objective was to regulate medical licensing, but it also sought to reduce the number of practicing physicians in the hope of increasing its members' salaries. Many of its policies were based on the 1910 "Flexner Report", a landmark assessment of medical education in the US. The gist of the report was that there were too many medical schools in the country, and that the entire educational system needed revamping and centralization. Specifically, medical schools with curricula not adhering to the "scientific method" were deemed inadequate for medical education. Important to point out that Flexner had serious ties with the then blossoming petroleum based pharmaceutical industry. His report was used to reduce the number of medical schools by more than half, especially the ones teaching what are now considered "alternative" methods of healing, such as homeopathy and osteopathy.[2,3,4]

On the demand side, wage and price controls during World War II prevented large employers from competing for labor based on wage rates. Instead they competed using benefit plans, the most lucrative of which was health insurance. The Federal Stabilization

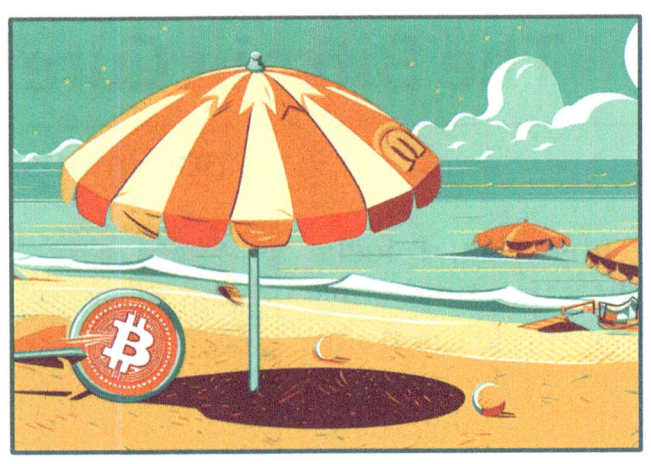

Act of 1942 made these benefits exempt from payroll tax, and ushered a large expansion in the number of insured employees (from 10 million in the beginning of 1940 to more than 80 million in 1950). Medical insurance coverage further increased by the enactment of Medicare and Medicaid in 1965. This is relevant because of a phenomenon called Moral Hazard, the tendency of insured people to utilize healthcare resources more than if they were uninsured (if it's free I want more of it). I see this often in my practice, when patients are given a choice between a cheaper test (e.g., X-ray) or a much more expensive and only slightly more sensitive one (e.g., MRI), they tend to choose the expensive one, as it costs them nothing anyway.[5]

The astronomical increase in demand due to mandated insurance coverage combined with a restriction in the supply of providers has played a large role in our current healthcare crisis. Patients are always seeking more healthcare services, but there aren't enough doctors to provide them. The AMA policies have succeeded in increasing physicians' salaries, but they did so at the expense of their wellbeing, as they are overworked and stressed about never satisfying their patients.

The most devastating effect of the AMA policies (in my opinion) is its suppression of alternative methods of healing such as homeopathy, osteopathy, naturopathy and chiropractic adjustment. These had their role in treating people before most of their medical schools were shut down by the AMA. In a free market model, the effectiveness of these methods should be judged by the consumer, not a central authority. If they are "pseudoscience" (as Flexner claimed) and less effective than pharmaceutical medicine, then the market will confirm that, as people would not visit these providers and they go out of business. The real purpose of the Flexner report was not the advancement of medical education, but rather the creation of a pharmaceutical monopoly on medical education (Flexner's ties with pharma are well documented). The end result: Even if ineffective, pills are now seen as the answer to all medical ailments, with no alternative.

In his seminal work of the same name, economist Murray Rothbard describes "The Progressive Era" in the early 1900s, which marked an expansion of the role of government in various fields of life. The state changed from an entity concerned with the protection of people's rights to one aiming to insure its citizens' economic well-being. That was the stated goal, but what actually followed was the formation of an unholy alliance between state intellectuals, big businesses and politicians to cartelize various fields of industry. Large business owners wanted to remain in power, and did so by employing "experts" such as Flexner to recommend government mandates. The fact that this expansion in government occurred around the same time the Federal Reserve was created in 1913 is no coincidence. A central bank allows the government to print unlimited amounts of money to finance its operation. In order for the AMA to have the ability to physically close down "unscientific" medical schools, prosecute unlicensed providers and maintain a propaganda so that the public remains oblivious they need large amounts of money, which the central banks will happily create out of thin air. The same applies for government mandates of health insurance and the financing of Medicare and Medicaid.[6]

Enter Bitcoin, a decentralized global monetary network that offers to revolutionize our economic and healthcare systems. Bitcoin allows direct peer to peer transactions without the need for a trusted third party. Therefore, large sums of money can be transferred digitally anywhere very quickly. Moreover, Bitcoin's finite supply of 21 million coins promises to make it the ultimate store of value for the future. A store of value is a currency that is expected to hold its value over time. The US dollar is a poor store of value because of continued government money printing devaluing it. While the physicality of gold makes it difficult to store and susceptible to government control.[7]

Bitcoin is the best store of value to ever exist. More importantly, it promises its users complete liberation from central banks and their money printing agenda. If Bitcoin were to become the global reserve currency, governments no longer have access to free money to finance their authoritarian centrally planned projects. Impositions that are not economically productive are unlikely to survive for long, as people (Bitcoin owners) are unlikely to fund them. In the case of medicine, licensing and medical education regulations would no longer be state mandated, but governed by market forces and what consumers find useful. A free market in healthcare could lead to the reemergence of more traditional methods of healing, and an era of unprecedented innovation in patient-directed care.

To conclude, this paper attempted to shed some light on the economic forces shaping our current healthcare crisis. The 20th century witnessed a massive growth in government jurisdiction backed by unlimited Federal Reserve money printing. In the field of medicine, this translated into licensing restrictions and insurance mandates leading to an unbalanced market. A transition to Bitcoin, a decentralized monetary system, promises to cut off the government's infinite money supply, limiting its intervention in the healthcare industry and allowing a return to a free market system. Bitcoin could be a revolution in modern healthcare. Whenever I have a stressful day at the hospital, I remember that we now have the technology to do better. It is only a matter of time before we transition to the monetary system of the future, and it starts with you learning and adopting Bitcoin in your life.

Sources

1. https://www.commonwealthfund.org/publications/issue-briefs/2023/jan/us-health-care-global-perspective-2022
2. http://archive.carnegiefoundation.org/publications/pdfs/elibrary/Carnegie_Flexner_Report.pdf
3. https://www.ncbi.nlm.nih.gov/pmc/articles/PMC3178858/
4. https://mises.org/wire/flexner-report-and-our-modern-medical-cartel
5. https://mises.org/wire/why-health-care-costs-exploded-after-world-war-ii
6. Rothbard, Murray Newton. The Progressive Era. Ludwig von Mises Institute, 2017.
7. Ammous, Saifedean. The Bitcoin Standard: The Decentralized Alternative to Central Banking. John Wiley and Sons, 2018.

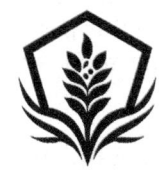

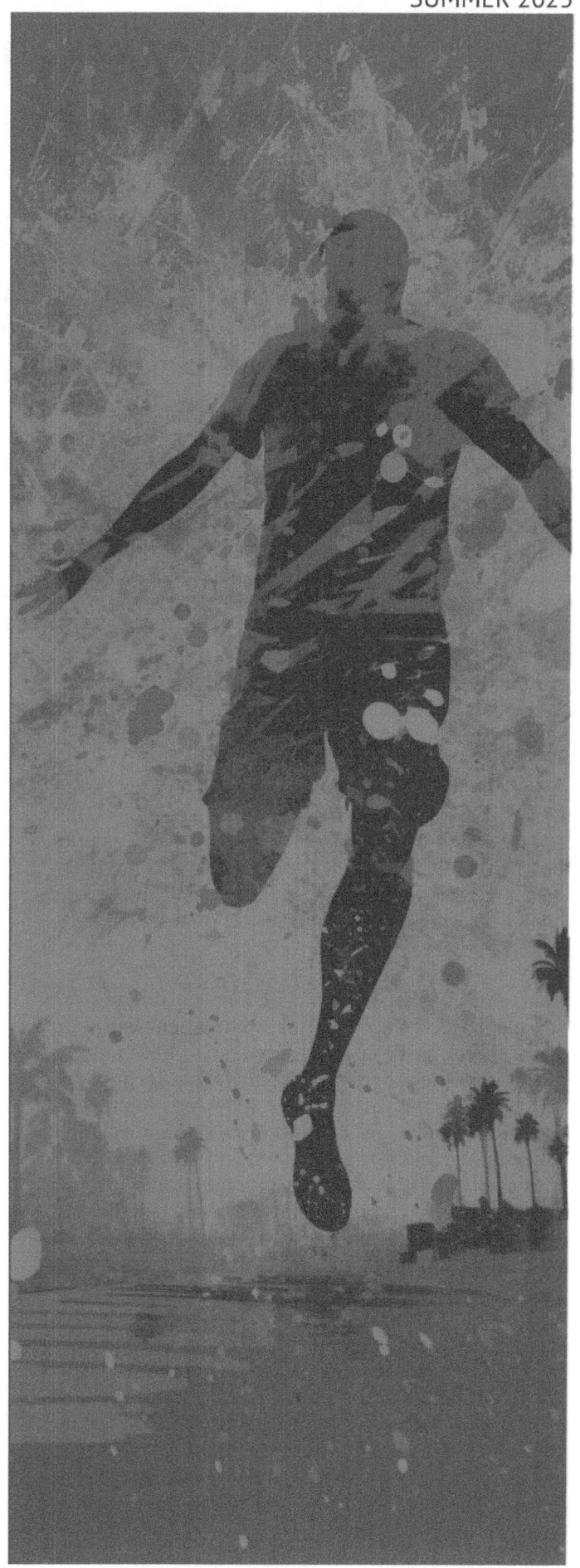

ISSUE 2 SUMMER 2023

What Is Value Based Care?

BowTied Tree Frog

RECENT headlines point to a breaking point with Medicare.[1] Rising costs of healthcare stem from Covid-19 lockdowns,[2] obesity,[3] and an aging population.[4] Will Medicare be there for you when you retire or qualify? Recent changes in how the medical industry bills may save us all.

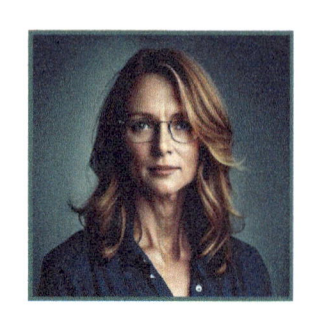

Value Based Care, also known as VBC, has been around since 1967; originally called The Patient Centered Medical Home (PCMH) it was designed to coordinate care for sick children.[5] In 2006, the term Value Based Care was introduced in Redefining Health Care.[6]

In a Value Based Care model, payments are tied to patient results instead of the current fee for service used in the United States. Value Based Care could be a solution for an unhealthy, aging population.

"The Centers for Medicare & Medicaid Services (CMS) defines value-based care as those programs that 'reward health care providers with incentive payments for the quality of care they give to people with Medicare.' CMS began emphasizing value-based, quality healthcare over the quantity of provider visits in 2008"[7]

What exactly does Value Based Care do differently? The model focuses on viewing each patient based on their specific diagnosis, using tools like patient education, efficiency, and data analytics. Technology advancements help companies quickly compile and sort data to help find opportunities to improve care. Being able to quickly analyze data and pivot to correct processes and workflows is vital for overall cost-effectiveness and keeping patients healthy. As more data is collected and processed, there will be more opportunities to improve care.

What does this mean for you? It will be years before Value Based Care becomes mainstream or standard. Once it does, you can expect to communicate more with your medical care group, have social workers to help find options in your community that could improve your quality of life, nurses visiting your home to ensure there's enough food and you can easily move around. The care would be tailored to your specific diagnosis and/or diseases.

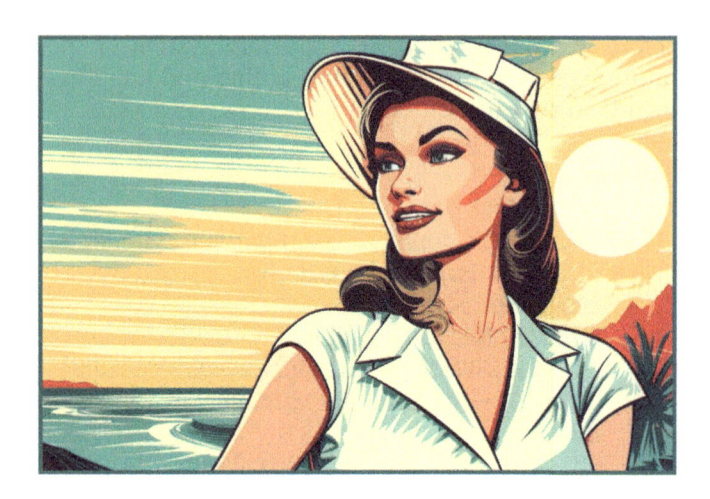

CMS aims to have all Medicare beneficiaries and most Medicaid beneficiaries enrolled in a VBC program by 2030.[8]

There are many aspects of Value Based Care that sound amazing. However, there are areas that will need to be improved before widespread adoption can happen. One of the issues that impacts the adoption of Value Based Care is the doctors themselves. Change isn't easy for some, and this particular demographic is stubborn; it takes time to convince them change is necessary and needed.

The most at risk for VBC are those in rural or disadvantaged areas; the ones who most require quality care. "... safety net hospitals and clinicians caring for poorer patients often get penalized in these programs. This happens in part because social risk factors are not included in the risk adjustment formulas that determine hospital performance on outcomes. Another reason is because safety net hospitals often need more resources to reach their quality goals, so financial penalties may be another barrier, rather than an incentive, to improving quality."[9] Fee-for-service doesn't provide the best service to these areas currently.

As VBC is tested and used, these challenges will need to be addressed. Everyone deserves to receive the best care regardless of location and local funding.

Sources

1. https://fortune.com/2023/04/26/ceo-of-cvs-warns-theres-a-medicare-tsunami-heading-for-the-us/
2. https://www.healthsystemtracker.org/chart-collection/how-has-healthcare-utilization-changed-since-the-pandemic/
3. https://www.tfah.org/article/nations-obesity-epidemic-is-growing-xx-states-have-adult-obesity-rates-above-35-percent-up-from-xx-states-last-year/
4. https://www.pgpf.org/blog/2023/01/why-are-americans-paying-more-for-healthcare
5. https://arcadia.io/resources/what-is-the-history-of-value-based-care
6. https://pearlhealth.com/blog/healthcare-insights/history-of-value-based-care/
7. https://www.elationhealth.com/resources/blogs/the-history-of-value-based-care
8. https://www.commonwealthfund.org/publications/explainer/2023/feb/value-based-care-what-it-is-why-its-needed
9. https://lowninstitute.org/value-based-care-has-an-equity-problem/

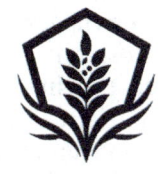

BowTied Tree Frog *is a veteran who uses her wealth of life experiences to produce a high volume of artistic output.*

You can follow her on Twitter at:
@BowTiedTreeFrog

And see her website at:
https://bowtiedtreefrog.com

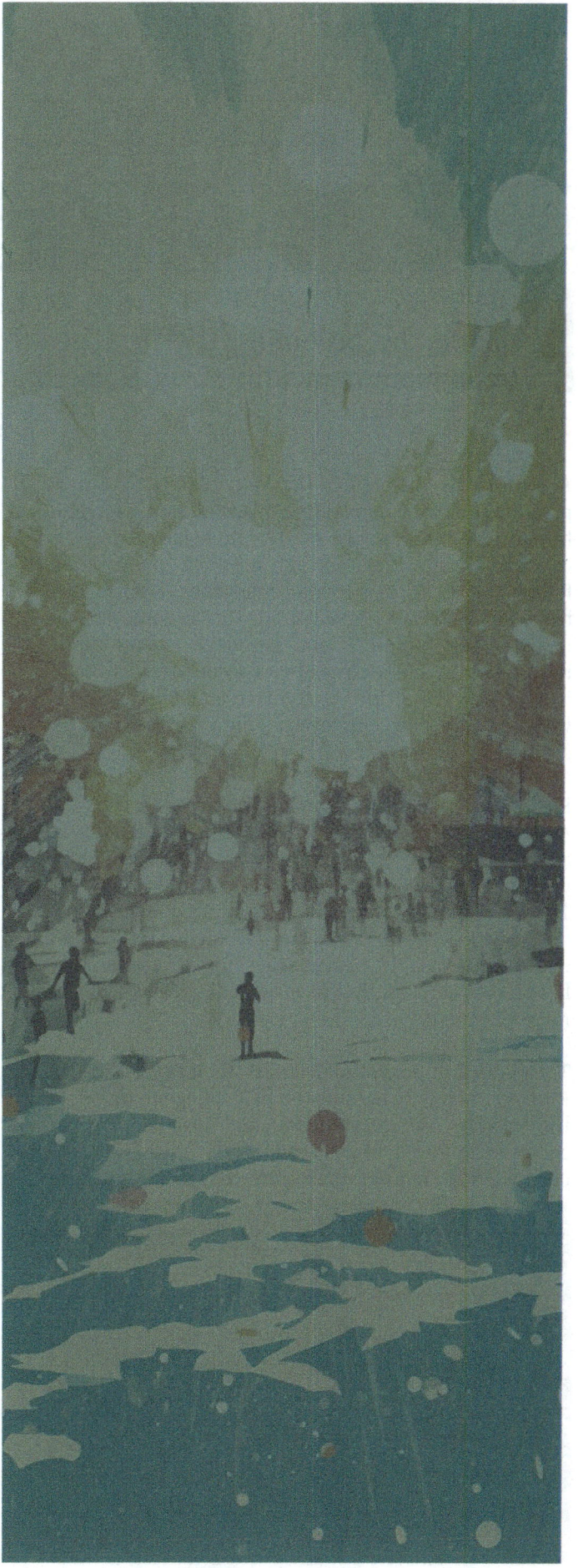

ISSUE 2   SUMMER 2023

Coercion Is Not Consent

Mary Talley Bowden

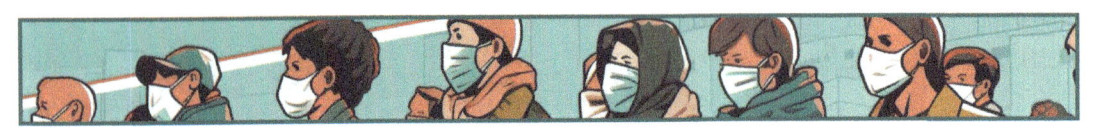

> **ON** March 31, 2021, Houston Methodist Hospital made history by becoming the first health system in the US to implement mandatory COVID vaccination for its employees.

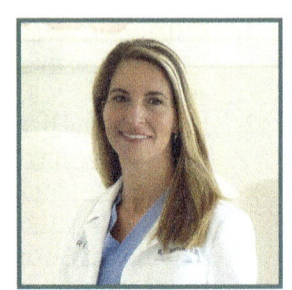

According to their CEO Dr. Marc Boom, "I think patients should be demanding this at all hospitals, and frankly, I think you will see the floodgates begin to open at hospitals. We've seen a bunch of hospitals follow suit. It took a couple of months, but they've been following suit. And I think you're going to see many, many more." As he predicted, many more hospitals followed their lead—a conservative estimate is at least 174 health systems mandated Covid-19 vaccines for their employees following Methodist's actions.

Five months later, the government followed suit; on August 24, 2021, the Secretary of Defense ordered that all military personnel must receive the Covid-19 vaccine. A month later, OSHA required employers with 100+ employees to mandate Covid-19 vaccinations, and the Centers for Medicare and Medicaid Services mandated Covid-19 vaccinations for all workers in health care settings that receive Medicare or Medicaid reimbursement.

The education system folded next. In November 2021, Rutgers University became the first college to mandate the vaccine for its students, and the majority of colleges followed their lead. Today, around 800 colleges still require their students to receive the Covid-19 vaccine.

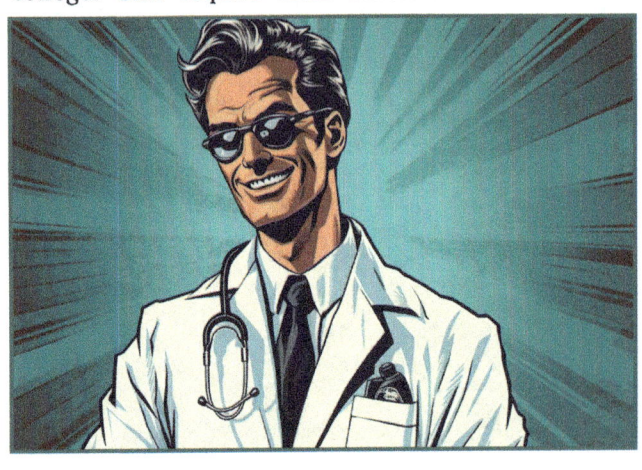

Lawsuits ensued; though some have succeeded, we still have students, healthcare workers and employees being coerced into receiving an experimental drug, still in Phase II (long-term) testing. The OSHA mandate was eventually reversed, but the Supreme Court upheld the mandate for healthcare workers. When the government ended the public health emergency on May 11, 2023, the mandate for healthcare workers ended as well. Some hospitals, like Houston Methodist, have chosen to keep the mandate even though our government has moved on.

As a physician with privileges, I was ordered by Houston Methodist Hospital to get the vaccine. Skeptical of the rushed timeline, I studied the data available on the Pfizer trials. Post injection, subject testing was up to the clinician rather than performed systematically; this was the red flag that kept me from going forward. I had also been using monoclonal antibodies to treat Covid-19 patients—with access to safe and effective treatment, I decided to wait on getting the vaccine until more safety and outcomes data was available.

My clinic in Houston became a busy testing center because we offered a non-invasive saliva test for Covid-19 with a quick turnaround time. When the vaccine rolled out in January 2021, I started tracking test results according to vaccination status. That summer, Houston saw a surge in Covid-19 cases, and from our test results, I quickly realized the vaccine wasn't working. In July, I posted this on Instagram: "We are seeing a huge upswing in positive cases, and unfortunately more than half of our positive cases are in people who have been fully vaccinated. The majority of these people also have symptoms." While vaccine breakthroughs were happening, I saw the power of early treatment (to date, all of my patients who received early treatment - over 5500—are alive.)

With time, I began to see patients with chronic and debilitating health problems following the vaccine; sadly I now see several patients a week with vaccine injuries. Backed by first-hand experience, I decided to forgo getting the vaccine and became more outspoken about its poor efficacy and potential risks.

Informed Consent: No Medical Procedure Should Ever Be Mandated

As a surgeon, I'm sensitive to the importance of informed consent and even published a paper on the subject during residency. All medical treatments involve risk, and a universally understood tenet is that patients should never be persuaded or coerced to undergo any treatment that involves risk.

Historically, physicians have held a paternalistic view towards their patients, but several court decisions have upheld the fact that informed consent and bodily autonomy are fundamental human rights. "Every human being of adult years and sound mind has a right to determine what shall be done with his own body..." In 1914, Benjamin Cardozo, a judge in the New York Court of Appeals and later an Associate Justice of the Supreme Court, was the first to hand down a decision that formulated the principles underpinning the consent model for undertaking medical procedures. Despite legal precedents, ethical standards and common sense, physicians in the last 3 years followed practices that blatantly contradict these principles—one cannot reconcile vaccine mandates with respecting patient autonomy.

True informed consent requires transparency, with discussion of the risks, benefits, alternatives, and unknowns. When the Covid-19 vaccine came out, the 'unknowns' were paramount. The vaccine package inserts are blank, and 10 year safety data is absent. Yet patients did not have informed consent discussions with their physicians or pharmacists prior to getting the vaccine.

Ideally, informed consent for the Covid-19 vaccine should have read something like this:

"This is an experimental drug. Since it is still in Phase II testing (the first long term testing phase), I cannot provide a risk-benefit analysis; we do not know the long term effects the COVID vaccine might cause. Death is a risk. No one can force you to take this vaccine, the choice is yours (or in the case of minor children, the choice is their parents). COVID survival rates vary according to age and co-morbidities; survival rates are over 99.4% for most people. Early treatment with monoclonal antibodies, ivermectin, hydroxychloroquine and other medications is an alternative. Pfizer studies showed an absolute risk reduction in contracting COVID of 0.84% after receiving the vaccine. Pfizer did not study prevention of transmission, hospitalization or death, severity of breakthrough infection, or long term safety data. Manufacturers will not be held liable if you suffer a complication after taking this vaccine."

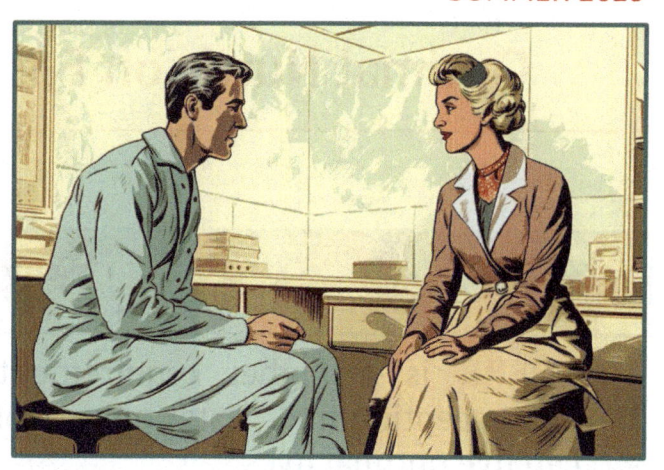

I've performed thousands of surgeries, and I've never bounded into the operating room without discussing potential complications—to do so would be blatant malpractice. I've never performed an experimental surgery, lacking long-term outcomes' data, but if we're to do so, I would feel ethically bound to discuss the potential risks and be particularly forthright about the unknowns. And if I were going to perform an experimental operation on a healthy person in order to potentially save another person's life, the risks of that operation would have to be exceedingly low—and the benefits exceedingly high—to uphold my oath to "First do no harm." Finally, not once have I told a patient, "If you don't let me do this surgery on you, you will lose your job... or be denied an education... or be discharged from the military."

Post WWII, hard to imagine medical coercion to this degree could happen. The Covid-19 pandemic unleashed the greatest crimes against humanity we've ever seen; the pandemic is over, but before moving on, we must process what has happened and hold the perpetrators accountable.

Mary Talley Bowden, MD *is a Stanford-trained Otolaryngologist and Sleep Medicine specialist in Houston, Texas. She has fought for patient autonomy and against corruption in our medical system. During the pandemic, she has successfully treated over 5500 Covid-19 patients.*

You can follow her on Twitter at:
@MdBreathe

And see her website at:
https://breathemd.org

ISSUE 2   SUMMER 2023

Optimal Nutrition For Preconception and Gestation

Ariel Acevedo

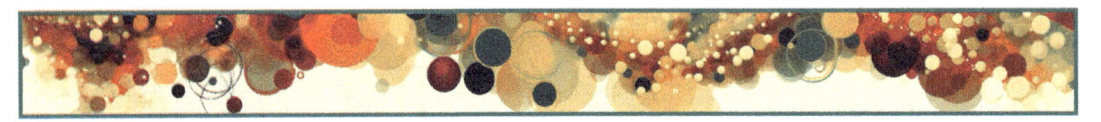

> **THERE** is a higher requirement for nutrients during preconception and gestation so both the fetus and mother can live optimal lives.

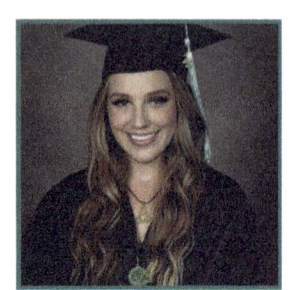

⇒ Choline is a nutrient that should be paired with omega 3's DHA. Choline works synergistically with DHA and is involved with lipid transport. Since our bodies can't synthesize choline, we must obtain it through a choline-rich diet. Liver, eggs, and red meat are preferred sources in prepping the body for future pregnancy. Choline aids the early stages of fetal development and guards the unborn against birth defects. Having a surplus of choline will help the mother as her nutrient stores become depleted as the baby grows en utero.

⇒ Zinc is pertinent for progesterone production and cell division as the blastocyst transforms into an embryo, then a fetus. Zinc surplus is connected to the follicular stages of egg production and mobility as it makes its way down to the uterus after conception has begun. Many fetal abnormalities began at this stage and dysfunction in cell division can prevent the chances of a strong implantation on the uterine wall. Oysters, seafood, eggs, and dairy are all nutrient-dense foods that contain zinc and are known to fuel fertility conditions.

⇒ Monounsaturated fatty acids (MUFAs) are also important for maintaining optimal fertility, as it is widely known to help regulate ovulation. I mentioned avocados as their nutrient profile is 66% fatty acids. A diet high in MUFAs lowers the risk of insulin resistance, hypertension, and obesity. This lowers ovulatory diseases and disorders that pose a risk for infertile women. Low-glycemic diets should be started before a woman decides to conceive for a higher chance of a healthy pregnancy.

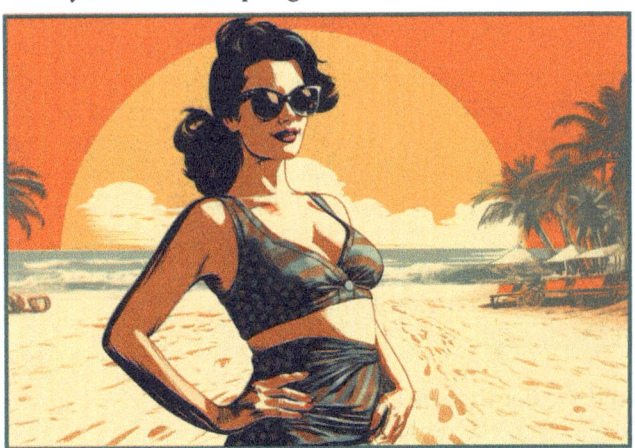

With the combination of these nutrients and living a proactive lifestyle, conception should come easily for most couples. Obviously, this excludes women with various ovulatory disorders or conditions where they are diagnosed with underlying reproductive system dysfunctions. Highlighting nutritional needs for conception is imperative for those who want strong, healthy children and a smooth transition into postpartum. The steps in becoming a good mother start with becoming your healthiest self, nourishing the body with the right foods will give your future child a jump start in living a healthy, desirable life.

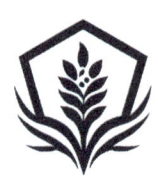

Ariel Acevedo is a student midwife and Everglades University alumni from Florida. She spent the last four years receiving an undergraduate degree in alternative medicine, using her knowledge in nutrition and herbal medicine to help educate women who are planning for pregnancy and a healthy birth. Her passion is in prenatal and birth education, advocating for women and their transition into healthy mothers.

Four Common Mistakes During Cycle Syncing and Menses

Ingri Pauline

> **BELIEVE** it or not, menses is a magical time. Like so many, I too used to believe it was "the worst" but honestly, I look forward to having my period—especially compared to the tension, listlessness, and the bloating the few days before it. A regular ovulation cycle is a sign of health.

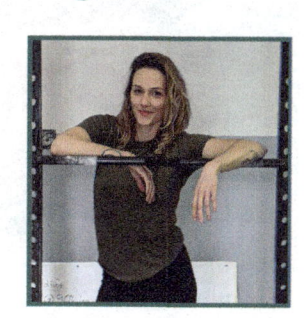

In fact, the American College of Obstetrics and Gynecology calls it our fifth vital sign. So if you are menstruating, count yourself as lucky and healthy.

Menses is not a curse. It's another phase of the natural part of life and growth. It is a dark and healing time to be honored and enjoyed. While the enjoyment we get from it is not the same as a good party or snuggling with our partner, it can be a time of bliss and profound presence; a time of release, forgiveness, refection, and healing.

If you ever felt you just needed a break for a day or two, your period is here to tell you exactly when you would most benefit from it. When I am in my premenstrual phase, I go extra hard to the end because I know I am going to largely kick back soon.

Let's go over the common mistakes made while cycle syncing during the menstruation phase.

Eating Salads
I get it, you want to eat healthy—but cold and wet foods are not the move right now. We still have too many women who think the only way to health is to drown themselves in green smoothies and salads every day. Apart from being not the only way to eat healthy, it will also make you miserable in the long run.

During menses and pre menstruation phases, our bodies crave comfort and warmth. This is the best time for soft, nourishing and rich foods. Soups and stews are great right now, as are foods that are rich in colors of blacks, purples, and reds. Baked potatoes and steak are good choices because of the iron and fiber content. My favorite food to make right before my period is any kind of black bean stew. I use meat and vegetables and sometimes some cacao powder to give it a deeper and richer taste. When served over rice, my tummy and mood are happy buddies.

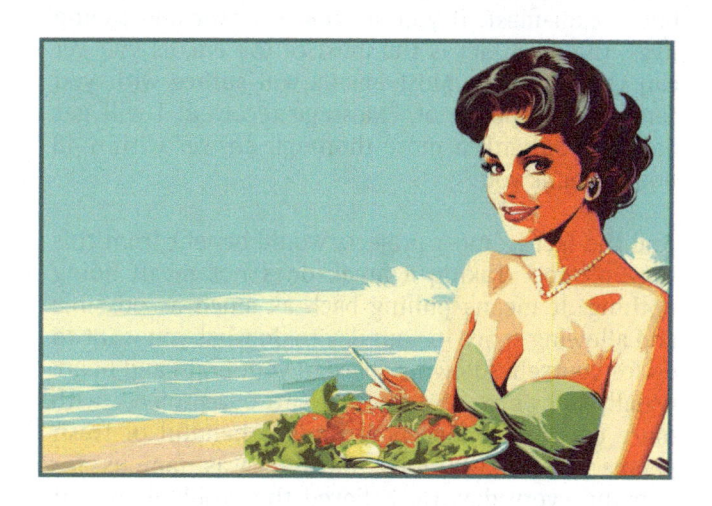

Rethink how you approach your diet around your period. Don't eat the same thing every day, and be mindful of this vulnerable and withdrawn time. Skip the fresh stuff and go straight for the warm and comforting food. This isn't permission to eat whatever you want, but it is a prompt to be gentle with yourself, and this includes your food choices.

Not Honoring The First Full Day Of Your Period
I see this time and time again. People want to get the benefits of cycles syncing but don't want to do the real dirty work and make the effort to plan ahead and pull back. So few women want to do this part—the part where you do nothing. They think they have to go-go-go forward at all times—but this attitude is what left you tired and cranky in the first place.

This Energizer Bunny approach is a good way to get an autoimmune disorder in your 30s and 40s. This is the fate of so many of the women that come to me for coaching. They're high performance women that are now suffering from their body attacking itself because there was never any space for rest during the first 15 to 20 years of their career.

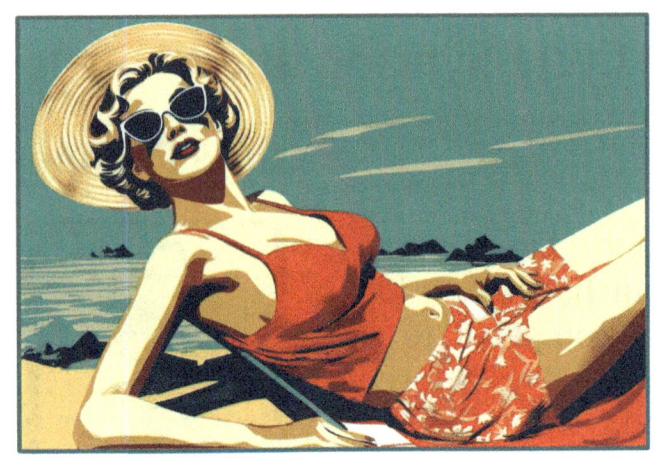

You must honor the first day of your period. If you have to make forward progress the very next day, do so but at half-mast. If you are not a doctor and saving lives, the hard fact is the most of the emails you get can wait one day. Most emails will suffice with you sending a response of, "Message received! I will get back to you with a more thorough answer within 48 hours. Thank you!"

And the fact is, most projects would benefit from this time off too. Taking a break does not mean doing nothing. It means pulling back as much as possible and allowing space in your day to do what you want to do for yourself. Allowing space in your brain and heart usually allows us to come back to our projects with more energy, creative power and a handful of fresh perspective or solutions. Einstein was famous for napping every day. He believed the problems would get solved in his subconscious mind. He is one of the smartest men to have ever lived.

This is where tracking your period comes in so handy. If you know your period is coming, you can prep for a couple of days off: do some cooking, tidy the house a bit, wrap up some loose ends or prep your colleagues to give you some space ("I'll have an answer by the end of the week, thanks").

ALWAYS honor the first day of your period. There is a lot going on in your body this day. Just give yourself a break from expectations and live in the moment.

Attempting Forward Progress
Sometimes we try to be sneaky and get some work done during our period and tell yourself, "But this NEEDS to be done," or "I'll just review what we have so far." DON'T do it!

The review process should have been done right before your period so that your relaxed and subconscious brain could do the problem-solving and heavy lifting for you. Right now your job is to pay attention to being in the moment for yourself. Reflect on your own performance and relationships with yourself.

Think about what you want to accomplish in the next coming weeks.

Don't fall down too far into the rabbit hole of thinking about goals and dreams, just set a small intention to focus on during your next cycle and go onto thinking about other things or doing things that make you feel in a state of presence. Read a book, take a bath, do some art, nap in the sun. Try to stay away from screens and social media. By definition they are the opposite of presence and they have a stress effect during this time. Take a day or three to unplug.

The purpose during this time is to get away from pushing forward and to just shed what is behind us. Even thinking ahead and setting goals is still putting internal pressure on our systems. Learn to relax with yourself and trust yourself that you do have the ability to get all of your important tasks done.

Skipping Recovery Work
Our bodies needs to recover and menses is the best time for it. Menses is a good time for bathing, steaming, massage, bodywork of all kinds, and gentle yoga. I just recently went a few cycles without focusing on my recovery and an old injury flared up.

At a minimum, the most helpful thing you can do are some self massage techniques. Using a tennis ball, softball, or foam roller to massage out your spine and large muscle groups is the way to go during this time. I like to plop in front of the TV or listen to a podcast with my yoga mat and balls and just stretch and massage myself for an hour.

This is also a great time to sleep. Naps, going to bed early, and allowing yourself to sleep in late is a choice move right now. You will be so thankful you decided to sleep during this time. As you know, the next week will move at a much faster pace in the pre ovulation stage, so getting rest to recover is your best use of time.

Ingri Pauline *is a women's weightlifting coach from Los Angeles, California. After serving in the Navy, she got her Bachelor of Science in Kinesiology at California State University Northridge. She focuses on all women's issues in fitness and health, including menstrual cycle synced training, pregnancy, postpartum and menopause.*

You can follow her on Twitter at:
@IngriPauline

And see her website at:
https://linktr.ee/ingripauline

ISSUE 2   SUMMER 2023

Biting Into The Truth: How Our Environment Shapes Our Face

BowTied Gator

CONSIDER your teeth. If you're not a dentist, you probably don't think about them much. Beyond our daily rituals of brushing and flossing, beyond the routine dental check-ups, our teeth hold profound insights about us. We're about to unravel a provocative truth: your teeth are telling a story—a story that challenges conventional dental understanding.

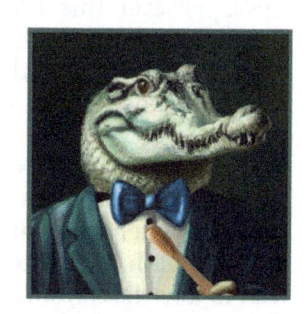

Malocclusions, retrognathia, and airway patency are complex medical terms, but they are intuitive to understand. Malocclusions refer to the misalignment of teeth, with Class II and III indicating overbites and underbites respectively, common problems many suffer from.

Retrognathia, a condition where the lower jaw recedes behind the upper jaw, is another concern that affects facial aesthetics and function. And airway patency; the unobstructed openness of the airway, which, if compromised, can lead to conditions like sleep apnea.

These dental issues are quickly attributed to genetics. Today, we're going to push the envelope. What if there's more to this story?

What if our modern lifestyle and environment, the food we eat, the way we breathe, are wielding more influence on our oral health than we've ever acknowledged?

My hope with this article is that we redefine the way you perceive oral health.

The Evolutionary Regression

We must begin by looking to our evolutionary past. Around 10,000 years ago, our ancestors took a monumental step: they switched from being hunter-gatherers to becoming farmers. This transition revolutionized our diet. The tough, raw foods consumed by our ancestors were replaced by softer, processed foods. This seemingly small shift eased the effort to eat, yet may have gradually changed our jaw structure, leading to smaller jaws and overcrowding of teeth.

Anthropological studies have found fewer instances of malocclusions and wisdom teeth impactions in ancient hunter-gatherer populations compared to their farming successors. It's as though the shape and function of our mouths visually reflect the echoes of our dietary history.

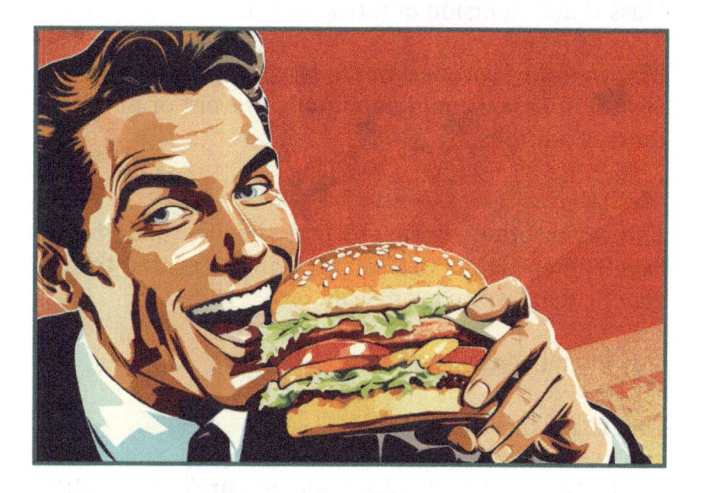

Fast-forward to the modern era, the dietary shift continues (except much worse). Ultra-processed, sugar-laden foods have become a staple. The change in eating habits coupled with early-life factors like bottle feeding in infancy, have been shown to alter our facial muscle development.

The muscle coordination required for breastfeeding is quite different from that for bottle feeding. Some research suggests that the act of breastfeeding exercises the oral muscles in a way that promotes better alignment of teeth. Bottle feeding, on the other hand, does not offer the same oral muscle workout. Could this early introduction of bottle feeding contribute to the growing prevalence of malocclusions and retrognathia?

Our propensity for a sedentary lifestyle is another concern. Physical activity stimulates the release of growth hormones, essential for the development of various parts of the body, including the jaws. When children spend more time on screens and less time playing outdoors, it affects their jaw development and increase the risk of malocclusions, retrognathia, and airway patency problems.

It's tempting to get lost in the multifactorial elements of facial development and forget the forest for the trees, however this becomes a vicious cycle. If the development derails from the beginning it can lead to a predilection for mouth breathing, which also affects the development of the face.

The role of airway patency in dental deformities is a subject that's gaining traction. Have you ever observed someone sleeping with their mouth open? Habitual mouth breathing due to obstructed nasal airways can lead to long-face syndrome—a condition characterized by a narrow face, open-mouth posture, and often, Class II malocclusion or retrognathia.

By promoting proper nasal breathing and treating obstructions, we could potentially prevent or mitigate these conditions.

Challenging The Genetic View

The association between oral health and facial development is no stranger to being relegated to the genetic hand we've been dealt.

"My mom had cavities"

"I have my dad's jawline"

No doubt, genetics do play a role in our dental health. However, the genetic argument is overvalued and a bit bleak. Despite similar genetic backgrounds, siblings can have different malocclusion types, suggesting that non-genetic, environmental influences are at work. Twin studies, which are often a gold standard for understanding the interplay of genes and environment, reveal that identical twins do not always share identical dental profiles.

Understanding how the environmental and behavioral factors contribute significantly to these dental issues, employing early prevention and intervention become paramount. The power of preventive measures cannot be overemphasized in this context. It's about setting a foundation for lifelong dental health, and it starts from the earliest stages of life.

Breastfeeding plays a crucial role in the early development of the oral cavity. It encourages the proper growth and development of jaw muscles, and it helps shape the palate. This can lead to better alignment of the teeth, thus reducing the risk of malocclusions. The act of breastfeeding exercises a baby's facial muscles in ways that bottle-feeding simply can't replicate, offering a compelling case for its promotion.

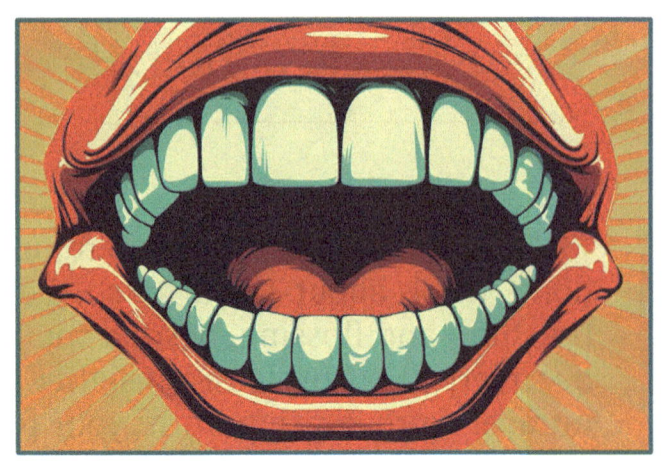

Diet, too, plays an instrumental role in dental health. A diet rich in whole foods, packed with essential vitamins and minerals, is conducive to the proper development of teeth and jaws. It's not just about the nutritional content, though. The very act of chewing tougher, less processed foods can stimulate jaw development, which could potentially counteract the trend towards smaller jaws and overcrowded teeth. Conversely, a diet heavy in soft, ultra-processed foods deprives the jaw of this valuable exercise, potentially contributing to malocclusion and retrognathia.

Physical activity is another important aspect. Regular, vigorous physical activity stimulates the production of growth hormones, affecting the overall growth of the body, including the jaws. An active lifestyle can therefore potentially help prevent underdeveloped jaws, malocclusions, and compromised airway. The modern, sedentary lifestyle, characterized by hours spent in front of screens, might be contributing more to our dental woes than we've traditionally thought.

Treating nasal obstructions and promoting nasal breathing from an early age can also be beneficial. As mentioned earlier, habitual mouth breathing can lead to long-face syndrome and other dental deformities. By addressing nasal obstructions early on, we can potentially prevent these issues before they become entrenched. This goes beyond the dental sphere, as proper nasal breathing has wide-ranging health benefits, including better sleep quality and improved cognitive function.

Another aspect to consider is thumb sucking and pacifier use in early childhood. These seemingly innocuous habits can exert pressure on the teeth and jaws, leading to malocclusion over time. By providing alternatives to these habits, we can prevent some of these issues from arising in the first place.

Early dental check-ups are also crucial. They provide an opportunity to catch potential issues early, when they're easier to correct. Regular dental visits can help identify and address malocclusions, retrognathia, and airway patency issues early on, allowing for more effective interventions.

The overarching message; prevention and early intervention are key. By addressing these environmental and behavioral factors early in life, we can potentially steer the development of our oral health in a more favorable direction. This perspective calls for a shift in focus from treatment to prevention, from reactive to proactive dental care. It underlines the importance of considering not just the genetic, but also the environmental and behavioral factors in our quest for better dental health.

A Broadened View of Dental Health

By considering malocclusions, retrognathia, and airway patency issues from an environmental and behavioral standpoint, we're not just challenging conventional wisdom. We're broadening our understanding of oral health and its intricate ties to overall health, highlighting the fact that our teeth are far more than just tools for chewing food or how we show off our charming smile. This very notion directly challenges the invisible lines that have been drawn in the sand by insurance companies that "dental, vision and health" belong in separate categories.

An Holistic Approach

I hate categorical terminology like holistic dentist or cosmetic dentist. Everyone wants a holistic approach, the same way everyone wants an aesthetic approach. However, the word "holistic" has value, despite its stereotype. I often imagine a world where it's typical for dentists to collaborate.

with dietitians to encourage diets that promote proper jaw development. For speech therapists to provide exercises to strengthen oral muscles, potentially mitigating the risk of malocclusions.

Even for ENT specialists to aid in treating airway obstructions, ensuring better respiratory and consequently, oral health. This approach transforms dentistry from a purely clinical practice to a multidisciplinary health service.

The Promise of Myofunctional Therapy

Myofunctional therapy has been gaining traction in recent years and is a promising avenue. To put it simply, it's a program designed to correct improper muscle function and habits affecting the facial muscles and tongue. This therapy has shown potential in addressing issues like malocclusions, retrognathia, and mouth breathing, especially when administered in children. Yet, it remains underutilized, highlighting the need for further exploration and integration into mainstream dental practice.

Personal Success Story

by Pastor Paul B
@PastorPaulB1

I'll turn 65 before the year is over, and I've been fighting an incurable blood cancer, multiple myeloma, since 2013. Ongoing, monthly chemotherapy keeps the cancer in check. This cancer begins in the bone marrow and weakens the immune system. If left unchecked, it damages kidneys and other organs, thickens the blood with 'junk' proteins while robbing it of oxygen, and eats holes in bones—that's the short list. At diagnosis, 80% of my bone marrow was cancerous and I was rapidly fading. There were holes in my clavicle, humerus, femur and 'scattered lucencies' (weakened spots) throughout my skeleton. My kidneys were severely damaged, I had lost over 30 pounds. I was constantly out of breath and weak. I remember choking back tears as I walked into the gym to cancel my membership. I was sure I'd never lift weights again—I could barely walk up the steps to my bedroom! Ten years later I'm in the best shape of my life, working full time and traveling internationally in difficult, high-risk places.

What turned things around? There was no magic fix or extreme diet, but I can't rule out miracles. Three things have been crucial:

Faith, which enabled me to face this battle with a positive attitude and gratefulness.

Great advances in medical research and new treatment options like immunotherapies.

A proactive approach to fitness, including educating myself on the scientifically proven benefits of resistance training.

I had been working out haphazardly for years, and my oncologist remarked that I was amazingly healthy for someone so sick. That seemed like a gross contradiction! I didn't feel healthy—I thought I was going to die. But his point was, I didn't have any of the common ailments that plague people who live sedentary lives and don't exercise. Lesson: if you maintain even a basic level of physical fitness, your body is much better prepared to endure and overcome when challenged with serious illness. I embarked on 16 weeks of chemotherapy. The cancer retreated so rapidly and I improved so dramatically with each treatment, the oncologist came in smiling each week saying, "We don't normally see results like this!"

(continues on following page)

The Interconnectedness of Health

Our exploration of malocclusions, retrognathia, and airway patency problems brings us face to face with the interconnectedness of health. It underscores that our bodies function as a whole, not in isolation. Our oral health is tied to our diet, our physical activity levels, our breathing habits, and so much more. Recognizing this interconnectedness is a step towards a more holistic view of health—a view that looks at the body as a whole, not just as separate parts.

While we're beginning to recognize the impact of environmental and behavioral factors on dental health, we need more research to definitively establish these connections and to refine preventative and treatment strategies. In the meantime, it wouldn't hurt to reevaluate our approach towards dental health. We must recognize the potential benefits of addressing the environmental and behavioral factors in tandem with genetic predispositions.

A New Era in Dental Health

In conclusion, a shift in perspective may ignite a revolution in dental health practices on a mainstream basis. Class II and III malocclusions, retrognathia, and airway patency problems are not just about being dealt a good hand in the genetic deck of cards, but rather how lifestyle and environment shapes our physiology. This is not to minimize the role of genetics, but to highlight the equally important influence of environment and behavior.

In this new era of dental health, we're not just filling cavities or straightening teeth—we're diving deeper, understanding the root causes of dental issues, and addressing them. We're not just treating symptoms; we're promoting overall health and wellness.

As dental practitioners, we have an exciting opportunity to be a part of this paradigm shift, to contribute to this broader dialogue on health. Let's seize this opportunity and usher in a new era in dental health—an era where our teeth tell a more comprehensive story of our health, influenced not just by our genes, but also by our environment and behavior. After all, every tooth has a tale to tell, and it's high time we listened.

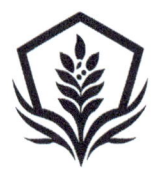

BowTied Gator *is the dentist that doesn't agree with the other 9.*

You can follow him on Twitter at:
@BowTiedGatorDDS

And read his Substack at:
https://oralhealth.substack.com

(continued from previous page)

Halfway through those 16 weeks, I was feeling better than I had in a year, and decided to restart the workouts. I was still weak and underweight, so I began with body weight routines at home: push-ups, air squats, crunches. After a few more weeks I returned to the gym, adding pull-ups, squats with kettlebells, bicep curls, etc. The increase in energy, coupled with muscle gains and improved mood, launched me into a new level of commitment to fitness. Scientifically proven benefits like increased bone mass, stronger muscles which protect bones and joints, improved immune function—these are the exact benefits that are keeping me a step ahead in the fight against multiple myeloma. These days, working out is a privilege, not a chore. It's the single best thing you can for your own health and wellness. If you put in the work, results will follow, and you'll be creating the foundation for a healthier future.

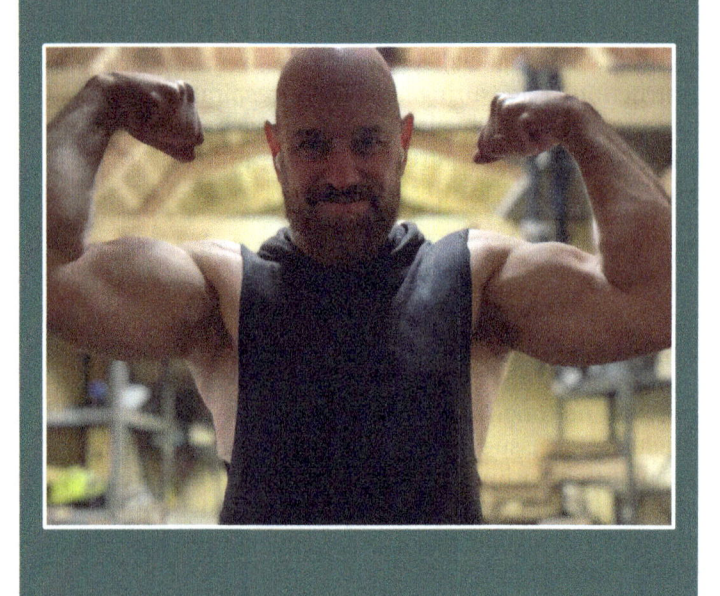

ISSUE 2 — SUMMER 2023

Crooked to Straight: Your Roadmap to Your Best Smile

Stephanie Steckel, DDS, MS

YOU made the decision to straighten your teeth. Congratulations!

This decision will likely improve the quality of your life in many ways, not only your smile. You'll learn how in the pages ahead.

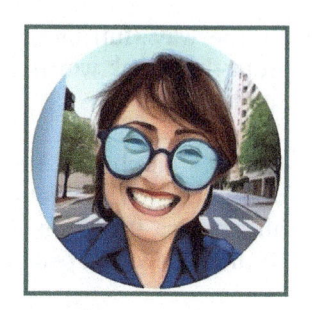

NOTE: This article is an excerpt exclusively for subscribers of Renegade Health Magazine from the forthcoming book "How To Prepare For Your Orthodontic Treatment, Handle the Process, and Enjoy the Benefits of Straighter Teeth".

Your Roadmap to a Beautiful Smile

You made the decision to straighten your teeth. Congratulations!

This decision will likely improve the quality of your life in many ways, not only your smile. You'll learn how in the pages ahead.

Over 2 million people each year—children, teens, and adults—decide to straighten their teeth.

They are teenagers who see their crooked or spaced teeth and feel uncomfortable in social situations. Or they feel that cannot bite or chew or speak clearly.

They are twenty-somethings (and thirty-somethings and older) who finally have some health insurance and disposable income to make themselves more attractive to others.

They are older adults who have wanted to do this for a while. They've waited to be sure they can afford it. (And with newer, nearly invisible braces available now they need not fear being questioned about getting a kids' treatment—Win!)

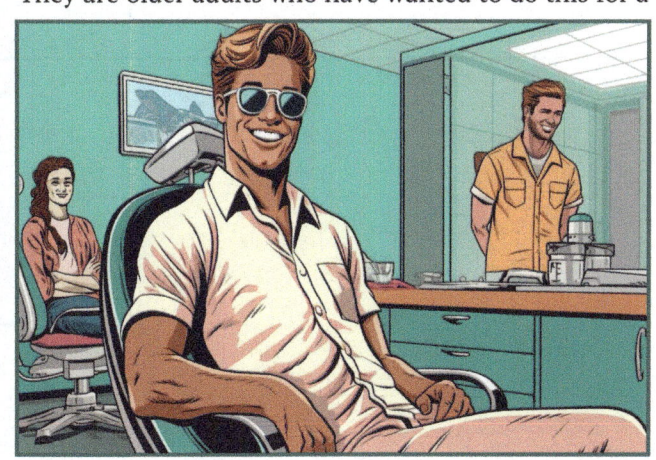

I have good news. People in their 80s get orthodontic treatment (assuming their gums and bones are in good shape). Even they can have the smile they've always wanted. (It's not too late.)

Why do so many people across so many ages get orthodontic treatment?

It's because a beautiful smile is an outward sign of good oral health.

Even more, it's a sign of positive health overall. Not just physical health, but emotional health too.

Research shows that "oral health-related quality-of-life improves markedly after orthodontic treatment, particularly in the dimensions of emotional and social well-being."

It's no accident that we often hear these words together like this: "They have such a happy, healthy smile!"

This is what people ought to say about you too. And they will after you have completed your successful journey to a beautiful smile.

A healthy smile is even tied directly to better financial health!

According to respondents to a recent study conducted on behalf of the American Association of Orthodontists, 75% of adults surveyed reported improvements in career and personal relationships after they received orthodontic treatment. And 92% of those respondents said they would recommend orthodontic treatment to other adults.

A beautiful smile is the most obvious result of orthodontic treatment. Other people are more likely to react positively to you and to your improved smile.

By the way (fun fact), the word Orthodontics comes from the Greek words "Orthos" = straight + "odont"= teeth.

But let's emphasize the fundamental basics of better oral health. When your teeth and jaws are in correct alignment, it means the function of your mouth (biting, chewing, speaking) is improved.

If you are one of the many people who suffer from speech difficulties, speech impairments, chewing difficulties, or sore jaw muscles, you might have been told by an orthodontist that teeth alignment will improve your situation.

This will give you even more reason to show that beautiful smile!

You can achieve the smile you want by doing the following things:

- Prepare for orthodontics in advance so you are prepared for the changes ahead
- Consider me your guide on this journey. (I am a dentist and orthodontist who has helped thousands of patients.)
- Select an orthodontist to treat you. This book will help you make this important decision.
- Use the roadmap contained in this book to guide and motivate you now and help keep you motivated throughout your orthodontic treatment.

"Orthodontic treatment is done over months or years. Make sure you pick an office where the staff are friendly and the doctor does the best work possible."

Pat B., age 38, former orthodontic patient and orthodontic staff, telecommunications technologist

Action Step
Write down the names of your current dentist, hygienist, and receptionist. Keep this handy with the office phone number. The receptionist can be a wealth of helpful information and save you time. Knowing their name helps get you connected when you call them.

References

1. 2019 AAO Patient Census Survey results at https://www2.aaoinfo.org/
2. https://kevinobrienorthoblog.com/orthodontic-treatment-improves-quality-life/
3. https://search.brave.com/search?q=AAO_Press_Release_Increase_in_Adult_Patients_1-28-16.pdf

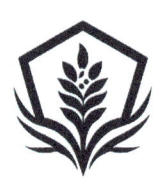

Stephanie Steckel, DDS, MS *is a Board-certified Orthodontist. She has practiced as both a general dentist and an orthodontist; and was licensed at one time in the states of California, New Jersey, Pennsylvania, Delaware, New Hampshire and South Dakota. She served her profession in several elected roles including President of the Delaware State Orthodontic Society and President of the Mid-Atlantic Society of Orthodontists. She currently teaches at Polytech High School in the Dental Assisting program and is a dental consultant. Dr. Steckel is a Burbank, California native and attended UCLA for her undergraduate studies and dental studies followed by the Medical College of Georgia for her master's degree in Orthodontics. In her spare time she loves to travel, volunteer in local community activities, and participate in speech competitions. She can be reached via email at docsteckel@gmail.com. Email her to be notified when her upcoming first book, Crooked to Straight - Your Roadmap to Your Best Smile, will be available.*

The FleX Theory of Power

Malcolm Flex

YOU are sitting in your room scrolling through Instagram (Not Tiktok, we hate Tiktok) and among the THOUSANDS of boring "Poast Fizeek" style photos and monotonous basic list of lifts people LOVE to spam, you see someone doing a cool-looking handstand from a basic press position. YOUR MIND IS BLOWN!

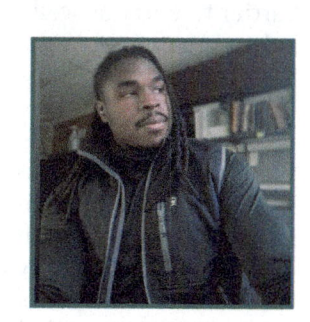

But even before you get ready to scroll down, the person then begins to lower into a push-up without their feet EVER touching the ground. It looks like it defies the laws of physics. You scoff to yourself, "Pfft, it has to be CGI." but a part of you wonders if it isn't. You then search "Handstand push ups" and you fall into a rabbit hole that would make Alice pass out from the depth of the drop.

THIS... IS... CALISTHENICS

Calisthenics is a form of exercise that uses your body weight as resistance. Calisthenics can help you build strength by challenging your muscles to overcome gravity in some of the most ludicrous ways. It can also help you improve your endurance, agility, and explosiveness. Calisthenics can also enhance your body awareness, control, and alignment, which can prevent injuries and improve your performance. Some of the most physically impressive (in terms of both physique and performance) athletes are Calisthenics practitioners. The best thing about it is that to begin, you simply have to master basic body weight exercises like Push-Ups, Pull-Ups, Leg Lifts, Crunches, etc.

Calisthenics can serve as an excellent compliment to a traditional weight-lifting routine or as a substitute entirely, offering a safer route to attain similar and in some cases greater muscle hypertrophy for beginners to intermediates while also building a greater degree of muscular stability and functionality. These come while also adding in a safer medium for making these gains, whereas untrained lifters trying to take their first foray into weightlifting may run the risk of injury or stagnant progress due to not understanding proper progression or rep ranges.

A few pages and article highlight the contrast and capabilities of calisthenics training as a proper stand-in for traditional weightlifting. (Also, you can do some cool tricks that can impress your friends. Probably not the ladies/fellas but we don't lift for them anyway, right?)

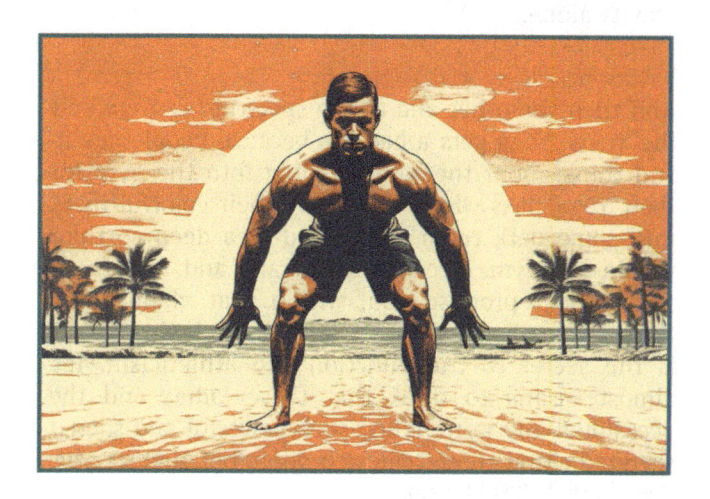

One study compared the effects of four weeks of progressive calisthenic push-up training and traditional bench press training on muscle strength and thickness in 23 healthy, moderately trained men.[1] They measured the 1-repetition maximum bench press, push-up progression, seated medicine ball put, and muscle thickness of the pectoralis major before and after training. They found that both groups significantly increased their 1RM and PUP, with PUSH having a greater increase in PUP than BENCH. They also found no significant differences between groups or within groups for MT and MBP. They concluded that calisthenics can be an effective alternative to conventional resistance training for improving upper-body muscle strength and thickness.

Another study was a meta-analysis (basically taking a look at the data points within a previous study rather than utilizing the framework to create a physical study yourself.)[2] This meta-analysis was done with a focus on the use of Elastic Resistance Training devices vs. conventional resistance training. (Elastic resistance training devices are instrumental when doing Calisthenics training as they can increase the passive resistance of holding what would otherwise be a static movement and limited in hypertrophy.) The analysis found that conventional resistance training offered no unique benefits in strength growth over elastic resistance training. Furthermore, the lower cost and barrier to entry as well as easy to perform nature of it led to greater averages of positive results though, at the same time, there was limited standardization in this analysis.

The use of calisthenics can be a game changer for MANY looking to either get started in the first place or switch up to a more well-rounded training protocol, as evidenced by the studies. It should not be neglected that sometimes the best weight we have access to is our body weight and the best mode of resistance is gravity alone.

The Special Sauce… Yoga

And then the other end of the spectrum is Yoga and the Yogis. Yoga gets a bad rap because people see it and think about the women going into the gym for their Yoga class where they carry their colorful mats into some dark room at the end of a deep corridor within the gym. It can seem arcane and foreign to some but I promise you, within that chamber of estrogen, artificially heated walls, and relaxing ASMR is the secret to true function and athleticism. It's almost insane to think that these ladies and the occasional guy were hiding such powerful and sacred secrets behind those hallowed doors but that's right. Yoga is truly THAT deal.

The more technical explanation for yoga is the ancient practice that involves the combination of physical poses, breathing techniques (very key), and meditation. Yoga can help you increase your flexibility by stretching your muscles, tendons, ligaments, and fascia (the sheaths and covering for our muscles). It can also help you improve your posture, balance, coordination, and range of motion. Yoga can also reduce stress, anxiety, and inflammation, which can affect your flexibility and recovery. Seasoned athletes will usually integrate some form of Yoga into their daily routine or training regimens either as active recovery day fare or as some sort of add-on to achieve a flexibility or performance goal.

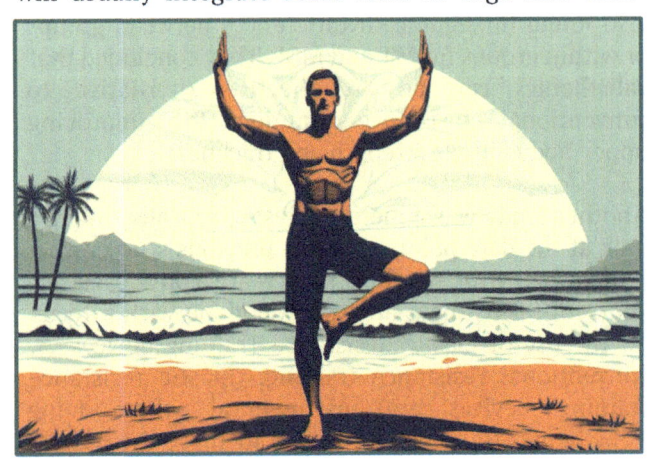

An article by Khan, Erlenbach et. Al cited the additional neuroprotective and extra effects of Yoga on the brain and how it contributes to positive aging through the usage of breathing practices, and postures that stimulate the brain, allowing for increased focus and attention to detail.[3] These effects persist beyond the duration of the actual practice itself. Breathing contributes to the regulation of mood and emotional regulation by improving the stress management of the body and building positive patterns. As a result, the addition of Yoga to daily training is a value add for non-athletes and athletes when it not only comes to performance but also a better quality of life. This makes it a perfect piece to the puzzle of a well-rounded life for anyone.

There are also articles showing the benefits of Yoga in terms of enhancing sports performance which is outlined by three articles in 3 different types of athletes along gender lines.[4,5,6]

As demonstrated, the benefits of yoga as a compliment to your athleticism are numerous and documented. There's almost no downside to incorporating some practice of yoga into your daily routine, whether you decide to go fully into calisthenics or not.

The Dark Horse, Martial Arts

For many people, I likely haven't factored in one thing that they're looking for and that's the "Competition" and "Conditioning" aspects of training on this alternative path to power. That's ok because the last piece of this trifecta is certainly not the least…. Martial Arts have existed as long as exercise itself for the use of the body as a tool for warfare is possibly the most primordial of uses of the body. Many people look at martial arts through the high-flying lenses of Shaolin Kung Fu styles although this is only scratching the surface of Martial Arts. There are so many styles of Martial Arts, let alone Kung Fu itself which simply means "Great Art" that allow a person who is beginning on the journey of becoming the fittest version of themselves to express the gains that they've made in either a performative or practical manner.

Most Martial Arts are explosive in nature or have explosive components to them that allow them to train the body to engage in athletic movements at high speeds, which can translate to greater athletic performance in other sports or activities or simply help an individual get better at the art. I don't have or provide studies for this portion as it can be tough because different arts can't necessarily be measured or compared to each other. BJJ, Sambo, and other grappling arts for instance have short-duration moments of explosion for which it would be difficult to test and make an objective claim but performance leaps in these activities indicate that progression is occurring in moves that require this level of explosiveness such as transitions, passes, lockouts, etc. These show that more explosive engagement of muscle fibers is being trained and improved upon. Regardless, you're guaranteed to get better at using explosive movements in rapid succession as your conditioning naturally improves and when you combine this with the mastery of breathing and focus gained through Yoga, you're guaranteed to go far and become an impressive specimen.

Not sure which art to choose? Explore your body and figure out what you're best suited for.

Maybe some of you want to become more proficient at kicking. Tae Kwon Do, Kickboxing, or Karate would serve you well, especially after working on flexibility through Yoga as well as the added core strength and balance of Calisthenics. Maybe you like the raw power of each of your limbs, explore Muay Thai, Lethwei, or Boxing. Want to get really technical? Go with a grappling art or even try your hand at one of the many animal-themed styles of Kung Fu. Like to mix and match? Go to an MMA gym and enjoy the full bevy of techniques blended or try the often misunderstood art of Bujinkan. (Ninjas rule)[7]

The options are endless and one thing that you will realize is that your conditioning will improve SIGNIFICANTLY over those who do traditional forms of cardio.

Getting Started on Your New Routine
I'm sure after being inundated with all of this amazing knowledge you're amped to get started on your new journey. (If not, go back through and reread this info and GET AMPED.) There are a couple of ways that you can begin training today. Many people, they're going to want to find a content creator or creators and get immersed into the community around the activity. Don't worry, I got you. Other people may want me to give them some starters and pointers to begin right here in this article. Don't worry, I've got you as well.

Let's begin!

Comprehensive Yoga and Calisthenics Communities and Creators
So many people want to get immersed and go into the community to meet new people and learn about what they can do to get started on their fitness journey. The 2 pages I recommend you begin to learn both Calisthenics and Yoga are as follows:

⇒ **Saturnomovement**. Saturnomovement is a collective project between Gabo and his friend Miguel and other practitioners of functional mobility. This is arguably the most comprehensive of the 2 communities that I will provide as they have tutorials that center around but are not limited to:

- Yoga Flows
- Calisthenics Skills Breakdowns
- Calisthenics Workout Progressions
- Core Strengthening Workouts
- General Flexibility
- Primal Movement Tips
- Everyday Morning Routines
- All Levels Training Seminars

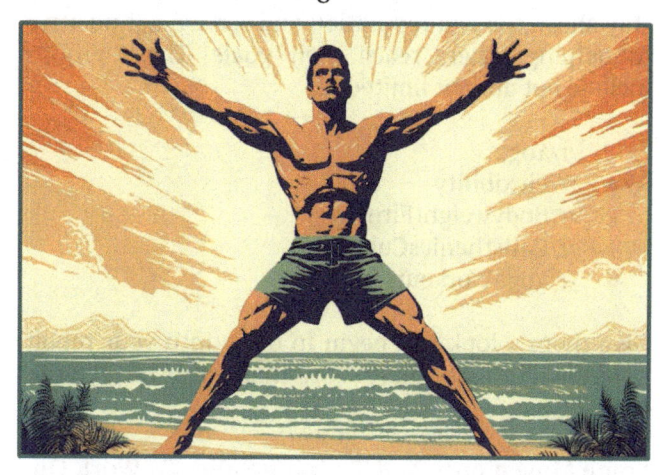

It really does make things a lot easier when you wake up and don't have a specific training plan. Almost any video that you find on their channel will give you some new ideas to train and work on. I can't recommend them enough to get started.

Some videos I'd recommend starting on would be:

- https://youtu.be/6Xw-OUcLp4s
- https://youtu.be/kN-yO7TShEw
- https://youtu.be/OCsxsGrFkF4

I could keep going down the Saturno Rabbit Hole, but for now, I think you've got something to give you a nice sampler and introduction to what they do.

On to the second channel:

⇒ **Fitness FAQs**. So this channel would be more for the people who would rather dump ALL their skill points into the Calisthenics bucket and are enticed by the ability to do a front-lever or a dragon flag rather than being fluid and flexible. That's perfectly fine and Fitness FAQs is like a one-stop shop for everything around the Calisthenics lifestyle. It is home to workouts, useful tips, podcasts from prolific people in the space, and talks about the science and methodology of Calisthenics.

Some useful videos which I would recommend for someone who wants to delve deeper into fitness FAQs would be:

- https://youtu.be/bn-HZm7bpy0
- https://youtu.be/TKYZTbyQQHY
- https://youtu.be/zqHhuHxtefE

Now, if you want to be one of those people that wants to mix it up with others, I would recommend joining some communities to get the full experience. This is where REDDIT comes in.

Redditors get a bad rap, but some Reddit communities stay above the bad reputation and serve a net positive to helping others reach their goals. These groups include but are not limited to:

- /r/Yoga
- /r/Flexibility
- /r/BodyweightFitness
- /r/CalisthenicsCulture
- /r/YogaWorkouts

Give them a look and begin to delve into your rabbit holes, as I'm sure you're more than eager to take the plunge.

Some Movements And Training Splits To Work On

For those of you who would like to take a more measured approach and don't want to simply splinter off into your own exploratory endeavors, I have some yoga movements you can work on and string together yourself, as well as a system to help you structure how you'll incorporate basic calisthenics training (See video tutorials or just stick with push-ups, pull-ups, crunches, and leg lifts). If you want more info on specific Calisthenics skills to train for, then that's where you're going to want to watch the videos recommended, as the approaches to gaining new skills and movements in Calisthenics is FAR too varied to be standardized.

Yoga Movements

⇒ Breathing. (Yes I know it sounds ridiculous but roll with me here, this is key to flexibility gains.)

Breathing is the foundation of ANY yoga practice and you should be sure to mind your breathing, keeping it at a slow pace through your nose at all times. Ensure that you breathe deeply, taking in air and expanding your diaphragm rather than shallow and frantic breaths. Some positions may be intense and the natural impulse will be to shallow breath but this will limit the amount of flexibility that you gain from a pose as muscle relaxation in a movement is KEY to progress.

There are different variations of breathing to try such as:

1. Ocean Breathing: The practice of constricting the back of your throat to make a sort of hissing sound as you breathe in and out of the throat.
2. Victory Breathing: The loudest of the breaths, highlighted by a deep and sudden exhale which follows a slow and steady inhale. Used to deepen your position in difficult poses.
3. Full Exhale: The emergency breathing where you want to go when things get rough. This is highlighted by breathing in through the nose and out through the mouth. Easiest to do as it's natural, just make sure it does not progress into shallow breathing. Keep your mouth small through this breathing variation.

⇒ Downward Facing Dog. This pose stretches the hamstrings, calves, and ankles, and strengthens the arms and shoulders. It also improves blood circulation in the legs and reduces swelling. To do this pose, start on your hands and knees, with your hands slightly ahead of your shoulders and your knees under your hips. Tuck your toes under and lift your hips up and back, straightening your legs and arms. Press your heels down towards the floor and lengthen your spine. Keep your head relaxed between your arms and look at your navel. Hold this pose for 5 to 10 breaths, then lower your knees to the floor. You can modify this pose by bending your knees slightly or placing a block under each hand. You can progress this pose by lifting one leg up at a time or bringing your feet closer to your hands. As an inversion, it can help your blood flow as well as build strength within your shoulders.

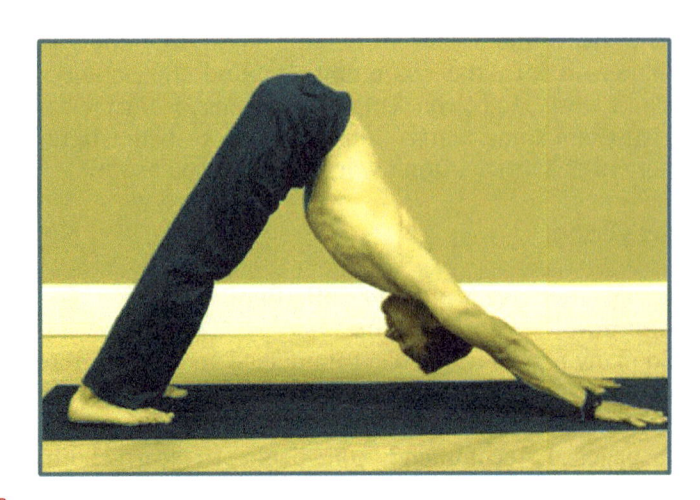

It's most commonly a stretch for the hamstring, calves, and ankles.

1. Come to your hands and knees, with your wrists underneath your shoulders and your knees underneath your hips. Curl your toes under and spread your fingers wide on the mat.
2. Push back through your hands and lift your hips and straighten your legs. Your body should form an upside-down V shape.
3. Press your chest towards your thighs and your heels towards the floor. Keep your head relaxed between your arms. Don't let your shoulders shrug up to your ears.
4. Engage your quadriceps (the front thigh muscles) and rotate your thighs inward slightly. This will help you take some weight off your arms and make the pose more comfortable.
5. Breathe deeply and evenly in this pose. You can stay here for a few breaths or up to a few minutes, depending on your level of comfort.
6. To come out of the pose, exhale and bend your knees. Lower your hips and knees to the floor and rest in Child's Pose, or move on to another pose.

⇒ Additional Yoga Poses:

- Hand To Big Toe Position
- The Warrior Series Of Poses
- Side Lunges
- Upward Facing Dog
- Chair Pose
- Lord's Shiva

Training Schedule Example

This is a rough example of what you can expect a regular training week to look like. Don't be afraid to mix it up based on your preference. If you want more yoga, then switch the Yoga and Calisthenics days around with more focus on doing Yoga.

Beware of trying to do both Yoga and Calisthenics together on the same day in the beginning, as your muscles may still be adjusting to the methodology. Take it at a reasonable pace.

⇒ Monday *(Calisthenics Focus)*
Upper Body Push Pull Work - Push-Ups, Pull-Ups, The specific training on a Push-up related skill like the handstand push-up or Planche. 5 sets of 5 for specific skills-based training.

⇒ Tuesday *(Yoga Focus)*
Choose 3 Movements and focus on flowing through them repeatedly. Begin to mix them up and hold each movement for at least 10 breaths. Do about 3–5 flows of these. Include Cardio or Martial Arts related training on this day.

⇒ Wednesday *(Rest, Recovery, and Relaxation)*
Stretching using some 15 Minute Saturnomovement Stretch Tutorials is also recommended on these days.

⇒ Thursday *(Calisthenics Focus)*
Lower Body based movements are recommended here. Consider Squats, Lunges, Jumps, and other movements that keep the lower body working. Bands are also useful to augment these movements. This is the only day when mixing in Yoga movements would be recommended w/ the Calisthenics workout. High Rep ranges here. (15 – 25)

⇒ Friday *(Yoga Focus)*
If you found the flows you've made were too easy, include more movements into them, 5 – 7 movements. Or consider using the channel and videos provided above for more guidance.

⇒ Saturday *(Calisthenics Focus)*
Full Body here. Focus on both upper and lower but omit the Yoga movements from the lower body as you're going to be doing a lot of work here. Add in some cardio to finish it out.

⇒ Sunday *(Rest, Recovery, and Relaxation)*
Same as Wednesday, maybe stretch today but the main focus is prep for the upcoming week again.

Conclusion

Well, that took a minute to go through, but if you're still reading, then congratulations on your newfound obsession. I guarantee you that's what this will become. Don't worry, you have all the resources you need and if you're wanting to focus on any of the 3 paths to power I've presented, don't worry, it won't hurt my feelings to know that you decided to discard my message of synergy. (Just kidding. Sorta.)

Remember that this is your path and it's simply an alternative to make fitness fit into your aspirations of being fit rather than the other way around. Go forth and conquer.

ISSUE 2   SUMMER 2023

Sources

1. https://pubmed.ncbi.nlm.nih.gov/29466268/
2. https://www.ncbi.nlm.nih.gov/pmc/articles/PMC6383082/
3. https://www.ncbi.nlm.nih.gov/pmc/articles/PMC4428135/
4. https://www.ncbi.nlm.nih.gov/pmc/articles/PMC4728955/
5. https://www.ncbi.nlm.nih.gov/pmc/articles/PMC7241641/
6. https://www.ncbi.nlm.nih.gov/pmc/articles/PMC4475706/#B51
7. https://www.bing.com/search?pglt=43&q=bujinkan&cvid=7065b87f315649bfaf6e4e0bbd036fb1&aqs=edge.0.0j46j0l7.2889j0j1&FORM=ANNTA1&PC=WSEDSE
8. https://www.youtube.com/@SaturnoMovement
9. https://www.youtube.com/@FitnessFAQs
10. https://www.reddit.com/r/yoga/
11. https://www.reddit.com/r/flexibility/
12. https://www.reddit.com/r/bodyweightfitness/
13. https://www.reddit.com/r/CalisthenicsCulture/
14. https://www.reddit.com/r/YogaWorkouts/

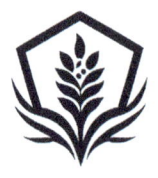

Malcolm Flex *is a 6'5 former D1 athlete turned MMA fighter, research expert, and honorary club bouncer.*

You can follow him on Twitter at:
@Malcolm_fleX48

And read his Substack at:
https://malcolmflex48.substack.com/

Personal Success Story

by Matt Izzo
@MattIzzo

The battle against excess weight is one that many people are dealing with right now. I know this struggle all too well, as I experienced two major weight loss journeys, losing 75 pounds each time, only to quickly gain that weight back again. It wasn't until my mid-30s that I lost 75 pounds for the third time but this time I kept the fat off for 6 years. The real challenge was not the weight loss itself, but adopting a sustainable lifestyle and rebuilding my self-image to align with a healthier me.

As a teenager and again in my 20s, I successfully shed the extra pounds but regained the weight when my old habits resurfaced due to life's turbulence. Demoralized by what I perceived as past failures, I spent my late 20s and early 30s numbing my pain with sports on TV, video games, and alcohol abuse.

At 34, I hit rock bottom and knew it was time for a change. I took a break from alcohol and, during a predawn walk, challenged myself to run a mile. That mile was a turning point for me. Stepping on the scale for the first time in years, I saw the shocking number of 234.4 pounds. Despite the initial shock, I embarked on my new lifestyle that morning.

I focused on eating less, consuming different foods, walking more, strength training, and daily weigh-ins. Within 8.5 months, I lost 75 pounds again, but this time, I didn't stop. I continued with my program and adjusted my nutritional strategy to maintain my weight. Month after month, year after year, I remained consistent, and my fitness also improved significantly.

(continues on page 72)

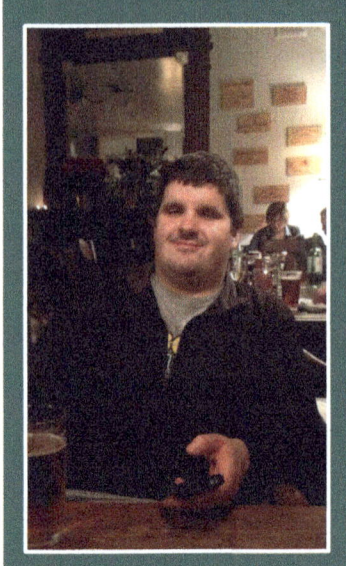

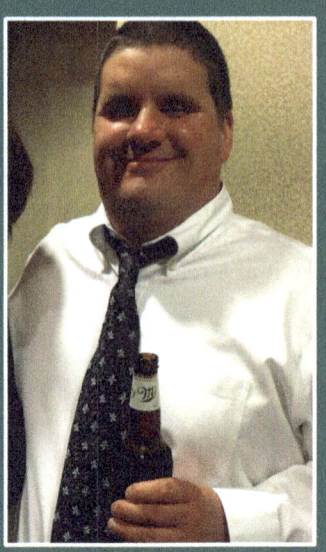

ISSUE 2   SUMMER 2023

Avoiding Back Pain From Deadlifts

BowTied Bengal

FOR every person that says the deadlift healed their low back pain, there's two people that got hurt doing it. From a movement pattern perspective, the Deadlift is considered a hinge pattern. If you've never heard of a hinge pattern, that's okay, it's definitely heard of you.

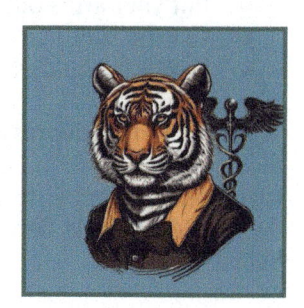

In a given day, you probably hinge hundreds of times a day when you sit down or try to pick something up from the ground.

A hinge is simply leaning forward and shifting your weight so you don't fall over. Feet on the ground and hamstring tension is what prevents you from falling forward. The "hinge" is at the hips, but you'll have some degree of the knees bending as well.

Powerlifting purists will poo-poo this info, but let's be honest – you probably aren't doing a powerlifter program. And their low backs probably hurt.

On a side note, back injuries with deadlifting can be serious, here's how to know if you should go to the emergency room:
https://imhurtnowwhat.com/back-pain-emergency-room/

How to Avoid Low Back Pain Deadlifting:

- Trunk Stiffness
- Pull the Bar Close
- Use Your Legs
- Make your body stronger

Trunk Stiffness

The first thing to reduce back pain with deadlifting is to know how to make your trunk stiff.

That starts with breathing.

With a big inhale, the trunk needs to get WIDER. You should FEEL the air get the low back.

If you have trouble with this a weight belt is a good teaching tool. Wrap it tight around you and be sure to feel your trunk expand into the belt in ALL directions. Then learn how to BREATH and maintain that pressure.

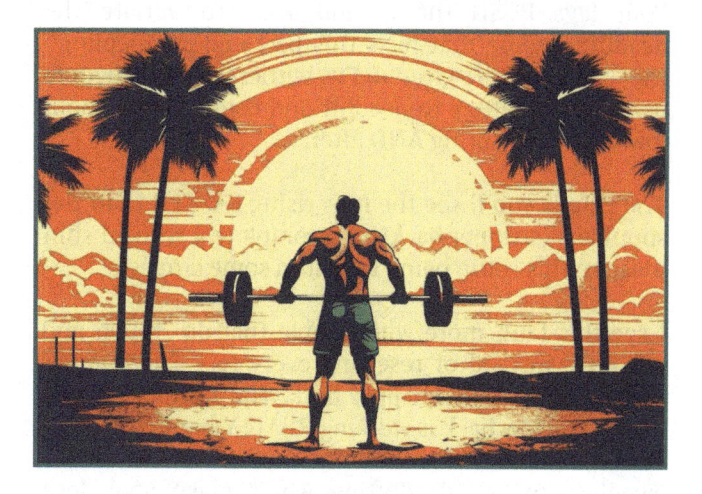

I have no strong views if you should use the belt for heavy sets or not, but you should know HOW to use it.

Valsalva
This gets a bad rap but it's misunderstood. Usually it's just thought of as holding your breath. To help, don't even give it a name. Just do the following:

- Take in a big belly breath
- Perform the lift
- Exhale when you know you will successfully complete the rep
- Repeat

The only change you make to your breathing is to WAIT longer before you EXHALE. In general, you'd exhale to initiate the lift or when you know you will be successful.

Pull The Bar Close When Deadlifting

The lats control the ENTIRE shoulder girdle. Use them to pull the bar close in the deadlift and reduce low back pain.

There are a lot of cues for this—bend the bar, break the bar apart, etc., the end result is to FEEL the lats engage. You should feel this same tension when you are leaning over, after you grab the bar.

To FEEL the lats:

- Put your arms out in front of you
- Get the shoulders towards the ears
- Get the shoulders AWAY from the ears

That's scapular depression. You will feel your lats. Most people try to squeeze the shoulder blades together. You may feel low back pain when you deadlift doing this because the excessive arch in the back.

Use Your Legs To Protect The Low Back

Your legs PUSH the ground away to initiate the deadlift. People that miss this part end up "peeling" the weight off the ground. I've witnessed many people using this strategy to deadlift and complaining about low back pain during AND after.

The clue is you'll see the hips rising FASTER than the shoulders (stripper back), or a completely vertical shin (despite this setup being taught in some circles).

I see this fault more with people that do "touch and go" reps, instead of resetting every rep. The bounce seems to force the stripper back. The "stripper back" means the low back is working REALLY hard.[1]

Needless to say deadlifting won't make your legs stronger, you needed dedicated leg strengthening and hip strengthening exercises.[2,3]

Stop Back Pain By Making Your Body Stronger

So above is all the technique and tension things, but if you keep hurting your low back deadlifting, you may have deeper, less obvious structural issues.

By structure, I am referring to the "S" Pyramid from StrongFit.[4] If you haven't heard of them, I recommend checking them out, but only if you like rabbit holes.

Simply put your BODY parts aren't strong enough to tolerate the forces the barbell is imposing on you. This means your low back will do more of the work with the deadlift.

At a certain weight, the deadlift is less a training exercise and more of a performance lift. Your individual body parts have to be stronger to PERFORM it.

The deadlift is a movement, so the movement will get stronger, but only to the extent of the individual pieces.

(continued from page 70)

In 2019, after reading David Goggins' book "Can't Hurt Me," I felt inspired to take on a triathlon. With no experience in swimming, biking, or running, I signed up for a race just 24 days away and started training. I completed that race, marking one of my greatest achievements, but knew I could do better.

My dedication to endurance training intensified, even as the pandemic in 2020 led to the cancellation of all my triathlons. Undeterred, I found my first marathon to run that year. In 2021, I achieved my goal of completing an Ironman 70.3 triathlon, and in 2022, I conquered a full 140.6-mile Ironman (2.4 mile swim, 112 mile bike, and 26.2 mile run).

The key to my long-term success has been a combination of physical, mental, and spiritual growth. Through thousands of hours of training, I have rebuilt my self-image as an Ironman athlete. This transformation was not founded on superficial affirmations but on the reality of my day-to-day life and actions.

Seeing myself in a new light has made it easier to maintain my progress and continue growing. Losing fat and keeping it off was a challenge that took over 25 years to master. Yet, I consider it my greatest achievement because it laid the foundation for everything else I've accomplished.

Addressing my physical health problems required immense effort, but it was worth it. My improved physical health served as a platform to enhance my entire life. This journey has taught me valuable lessons about perseverance, self-discovery, and the importance of a holistic approach to health and well-being. My transformation is a testament to the power of dedication and the belief that it's never too late to make a positive change.

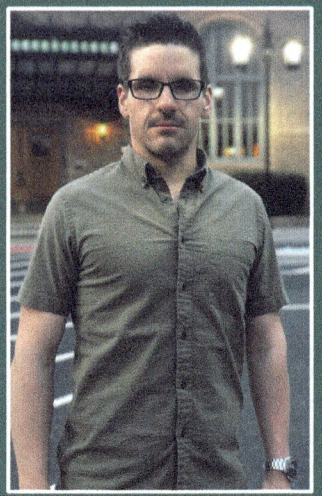

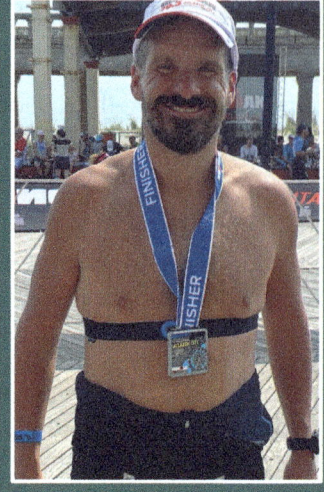

A 135lb deadlift is a COMPLETELY different movement than a 405lbs. (and UP) deadlift.

What's this mean? As the bar gets heavier, it also gets LONGER. The distance from 1 to 2 is 26 inches, and 2 to 3 is 16 inches. So, 1 plate versus ALL the plates is 40% more length added to the bar, PLUS the bar in bending.

The deadlift is literally trying to rip you (low back and all) apart. Your structure HAS to be able to withstand this.

Based on that, I'm a fan of StrongFit's structural strength recommendations, which are:

- 50 m sandbag carry 50% of 1rm.[5]
- 20 m farmers carry 100% of 1rm split between each hand.[6]
- 5x barbell/dumbbell row 50%/30% of 1rm.

This starts to get into the realm of specialization for the deadlift, so basically you deadlift because you compete. Competing means you accept the risk of back pain.

Not meeting this doesn't mean don't deadlift, but working towards this is a great way to decrease the risk of experiencing low back pain with the deadlift.

Summary

Hurting your low back while deadlifting is totally unnecessary if you are just a casual strength trainee focused on general fitness. And these tips will definitely help you out. At the end of the day, a good training program is the most protective against injury.

Sources

1. https://youtu.be/Y6aHiKvs7Do
2. https://imhurtnowwhat.com/best-exercises-for-knee-pain/
3. https://imhurtnowwhat.com/hip-strength-exercises/
4. https://www.instagram.com/strongfit1/
5. https://www.youtube.com/watch?v=vUlN6Hz0vv0&t=21s
6. https://www.youtube.com/watch?v=U1Sbv0ZTKG0&t=234s

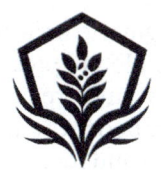

BowTied Bengal *is a doctor of physical therapy with a decade of experience in orthopedics and sports medicine, and spent many years treating the spine and chronic pain. He also knows his way around a weight room as most of his continuing education comes from the world of strength and conditioning. That experience makes him an expert in working around an injury as well as the long term management of chronic conditions. Being a patient sucks, so his goal is to get you out of that phase ASAP and back to doing the things you love.*

You can follow him on Twitter at:
@BowTied_Bengal

And read his articles at:
https://imhurtnowwhat.com

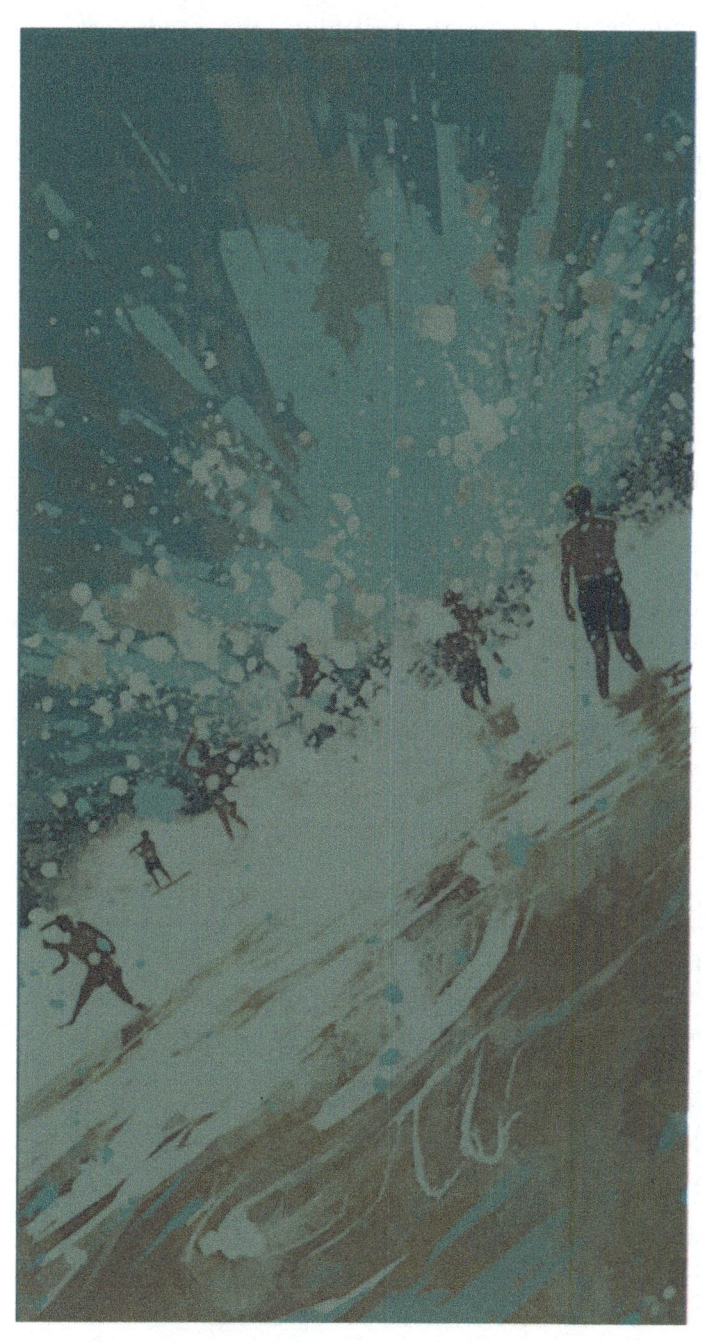

Breathe Your Way To Better Health

Brian The Beard

DIAPHRAGMATIC breathing used to be innate within us as human beings—it has now become almost a forgotten language to us. Societal advances and technology have drawn our attention to the outside world, causing us to lose complete awareness of our bodily functions.

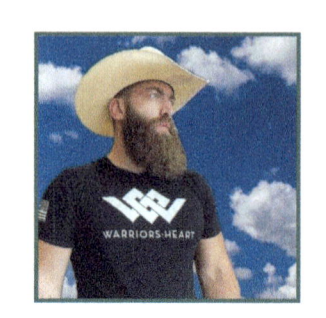

Without diaphragmatic breathing, our respiratory system, cardiovascular system, musculoskeletal system, digestive system, and nervous system cannot function at 100% efficiency. Therefore, it is important to relearn this breathing technique to ensure that all our bodily systems are functioning optimally.

The dissociation of these bodily systems will inevitably lead to minor and major health issues throughout an individual's life. It is therefore crucial to prevent these health issues by understanding what diaphragmatic breathing is and how to practice it.

How The Diaphragm Works

Diaphragmatic breathing is characterized by a deep, slow, and rhythmic pattern of breathing in which the torso expands and contracts with each breath, rather than the chest. This breathing technique involves using the diaphragm, a large muscle located between the chest and the abdomen, to control the inhalation and exhalation of air.

During diaphragmatic breathing when you inhale, your diaphragm contracts and moves downward, allowing the lungs to expand and fill with oxygen. When you exhale, the diaphragm relaxes and ascends, helping to push air out of the lungs. Practicing this technique ensures that your body is receiving the proper amount of oxygen and that all your bodily systems are functioning optimally.

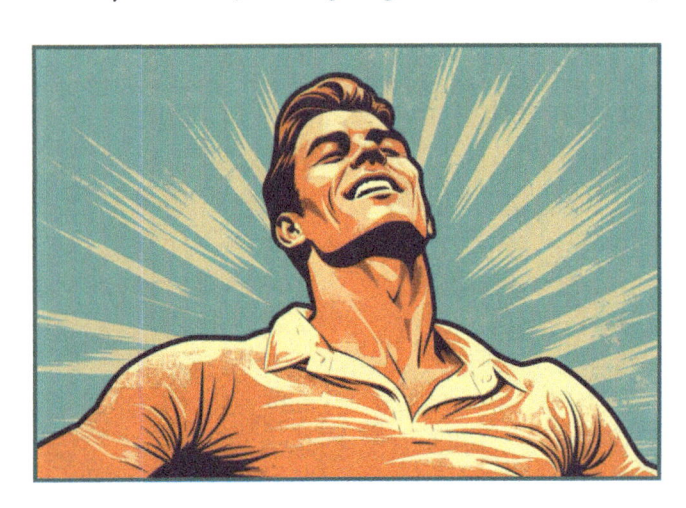

Proper breathing allows the lungs to work their magic, exchanging carbon dioxide for oxygen and helping to maintain balance in cellular metabolism, along with other physiological processes.

Now that we understand what diaphragmatic breathing is and how it works, let's discuss how to access the diaphragm.

The respiratory system begins and ends at the nostrils. The pathway for natural respiratory mechanics runs through the nasal passages and allows the diaphragm to complete the respiratory cycle. Focusing on breathing through the nose and using the diaphragm to control inhalation and exhalation, you can ensure that you are practicing diaphragmatic breathing correctly and reaping its benefits.

Alleviating Stress

Stress can significantly impact your quality of life, affecting you physically, emotionally, cognitively, and behaviorally. Having full control over your autonomic nervous system through proper breathing is one of the best life hacks out there. By breathing deeply from the diaphragm, you can activate the parasympathetic nervous system, which helps to counteract the fight or flight response that is activated during times of anxiety and mental or physical stress.

By practicing diaphragmatic breathing you can reduce stress levels, lower blood pressure, and increase feelings of calmness and relaxation. It can also improve sleep quality, boost the immune system, and enhance mental clarity and focus.

Managing Pain

Diaphragmatic breathing can also be a useful tool for managing pain. This technique can alleviate pain caused by muscle tension or spasm and promote relaxation throughout the body. For example, applying trigger point therapy on fascia can be enhanced by diaphragmatic breathing. When working on a particular knot, an exaggerated exhale can help to relieve the pain and even remove the knot.

Improving Posture

By inhibiting bodily pain, you can improve your posture, mobility, and blood circulation, ultimately leading to a better quality of life. Practicing diaphragmatic breathing regularly can help you manage chronic pain, reduce inflammation, and enhance your overall physical and mental well-being. So, take a deep breath, focus on your diaphragm, and experience the benefits of this simple yet powerful technique.

Inhaling through the mouth can cause the chest to expand and contract the pectoralis major and minor muscles, leading to a rise in the shoulders. This can have a direct impact on your posture and it is a common problem in today's world.

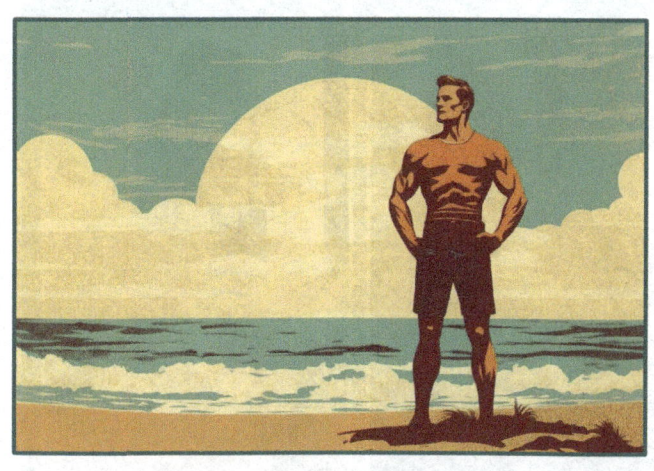

Furthermore, fascia can harden around supporting muscles, bones, and organs during times of stress. As a highly innervated tissue, fascia responds to changes in the body including changes in stress levels. This can restrict an individual's movement patterns, increase bodily pain and discomfort, and hinder exercise efficiency.

Improving Sleep

Poor breathing patterns can have a close association with sleep apnea, insomnia, and restless leg syndrome which you or a friend may be suffering from. Incorrect breathing throughout sleep can significantly affect its quality and duration, leading to the development of these sleep disorders. While there are various factors that contribute to poor sleep quality, proper breathing is the most crucial aspect to address.

Diaphragmatic breathing can promote relaxation to reduce bodily tension, lower blood pressure, increase oxygen intake, and regulate the nervous system. By practicing proper breathing techniques, you can take control of your sleep and improve its quality, leading to better overall health and well-being.

Rediscover Your Diaphragm

Rediscovering how to breathe correctly is not accomplished in a day. It will take repetitions to make this new breathing pattern, your daily habit. The basics of finding your diaphragm through the breath takes only a couple of steps.

- Make sure your rib cage is stacked over your hips
- Nasal Breathe
- Don't breathe with a fast or heavy cadence

Now, these steps can be read simply but each and every individual is unique. We all have our own compensations that do hold us back from easily accomplishing this feat, in our natural posture.

Crocodile Breathing

Whether you know if you are capable of performing a deep breath or not, I recommend all readers to try this exercise:

- Lie on your stomach with your hands by your sides and your forehead resting on the floor
- If the front of your hips are hanging off the ground, imagine pulling your hips to the bottom of your rib cage (This is a temporary stacked position)
- Take a subtle 3-second inhale through your nose and into the bottom of your lungs
- Hold that breath for 3 good seconds
- Feel the expansion in your torso and rib cage
- Slowly exhale through the mouth for 6 seconds
- Feel the relaxation throughout the body
- Start the process over again

Diaphragmatic breathing is an essential tool for achieving optimal health and well-being. By learning to breathe from the diaphragm, we can reduce stress and anxiety, manage pain, and promote better sleep. Deep breathing is a simple and effective way to promote relaxation and balance in our bodies, allowing us to face the challenges of daily life. With regular practice and mindfulness, diaphragmatic breathing can become a natural and effortless part of our daily routine, helping us to live happier, healthier lives.

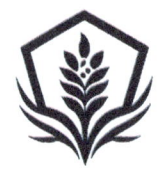

Brian The Beard *was born with a rare seizure disorder, had low self esteem, and lacked confidence in the weight room. Now, 20 years later, he conquered those limitations and is now a full time Personal Trainer in Austin, Texas. He specializes in breathwork, strength training and PRI protocols. He trains clients from big name CEOs to the average joe.*

You can follow him on Twitter at:
@Brian_Venturino

And see his website at:
https://breathingforexcellence.carrd.co

Personal Success Story

by Catherine

I am a 42-year-old mother and wife. I changed my entire life. Like most people I didn't have a great relationship with food. I ate when I was happy to celebrate, when I was sad for the comfort. Sometimes I even mindlessly ate.

I had gotten so large 400lbs I was losing my ability to walk, I was devastated. 2015 I was told if I didn't change I would be dead in a year.

I remember something changed for me I said, "no I won't." I made little changes cut out soda, I even used a child's plate for portion control. I found free videos on YouTube and I worked out 3 times a week.

The NSV (non scale victories) led to me loving what I was doing. I kept showing up for myself every day.

I am now 150lbs I am pretty muscular because of my success I have helped many people lose weight. I offer my support and my guidance. I hope to inspire people to be success stories.

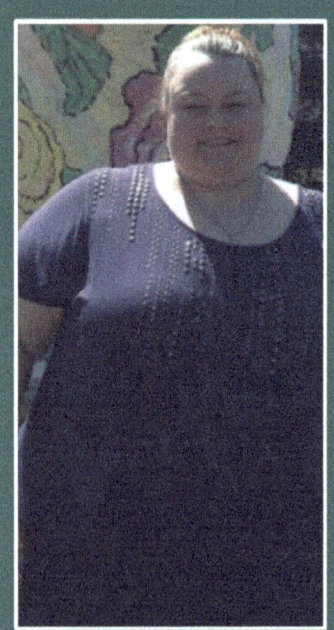

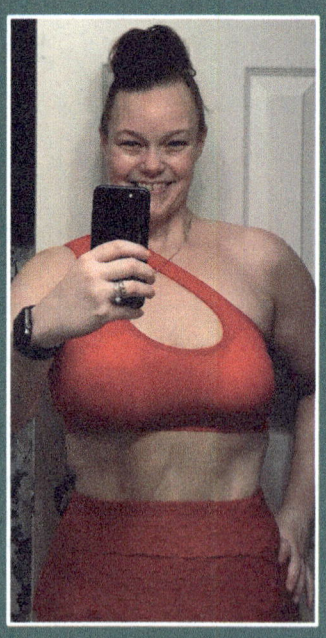

Conquer Your Sleep Disorder: Part II

BowTied Hermit Crab

OUR previous article *(see Renegade Health Magazine Issue 1 Spring 2023)* discussed the pathways towards a sleep apnea diagnosis. We reviewed the different pathways— home-based versus attended in-center. Then we reviewed copays and deductibles, and how they apply to sleep testing.

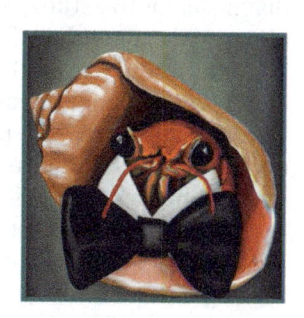

Many of the billing concepts covered in the previous article remain true for all healthcare diagnostic testing. In this article we will build on the foundation from the diagnostic pathway and get to the data review. We are going to cover everything from acronyms to numbers and terms to a diagnosis.

The Home Sleep Apnea Test (HSAT) can resemble different aesthetics these days compared to a number of years ago. There are some devices that go on the finger, wrap around the wrist, patch-type sensors, and belt/flow devices. The attended in-lab polysomnogram (PSG) has standards of setup and categories of equipment to be used. Either way, the American Academy of Sleep Medicine requires that studies use standards when reporting data. The most important data points or standard reporting metrics, as related strictly to sleep apnea and according to the American Academy of Sleep Medicine (AASM)[1] are the following.

Apnea-Hypopnea Index (AHI)
Typically seen on PSG studies and is determined by the number of apneas plus the number of hypopneas x 60 divided by total sleep time (TST).

Respiratory Event Index (REI)
Required to be reported on a HSAT; number of apneas plus the number of hypopneas x60 divided by MT.

Respiratory Disturbance Index (RDI)
Seen on PSG studies and is determined by the number of apneas plus the number of hypopneas plus the number of respiratory effort-related arousals (RERA) x60 divided by total sleep time; this number is important because these are events that are directly causing arousals but may not be classic apnea/hypopneas.

Monitoring Time (MT)
Reported on HSAT; data adequate for interpretation/analysis.

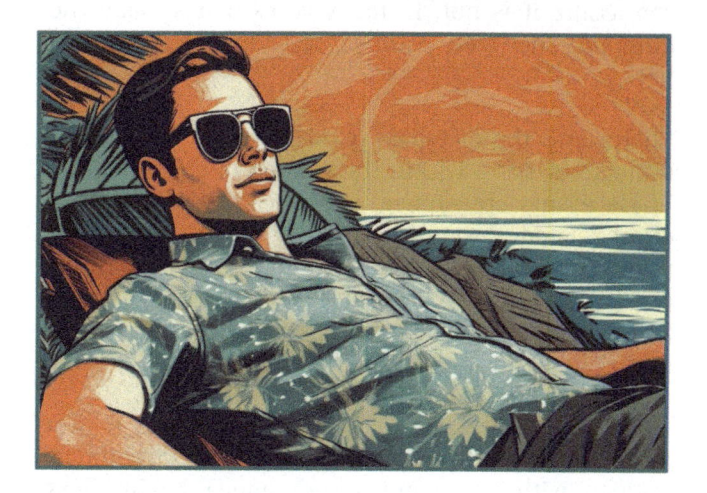

Recording Time (RT)
Total data/duration recorded; not necessarily adequate but includes MT as well.

Total Sleep Time (TST)
The PSG equivalent of MT above.

The data points mentioned above all create a number of important chart elements for every study and paint the picture of a patient's sleep architecture. They are.

Histogram/Hypnogram
This is a timeline and a summation, in graphical terms, of all events that occurred during the study. You can see colored-lines for color-coded event types, positional changes, heart rate, pulse oximetry, limb movements, et al. This gives your provider the entire study in one image.

Raw data printouts
The raw data is typically the numerical analysis that generated all the lines and bars above. This is the part where the acronyms mentioned come into play. There is a wealth of information in the raw data that, at times, may not make it into the final report. These documents may contain a treasure trove of

information to personalize care when compared to just having the final report (interpretation).

Interpretation
The final report is a document that includes a final diagnosis for the study, impression, recommendations, along with some data from the raw data report, any abnormalities in the electrocardiogram and electroencephalogram, and scoring definition utilized. Unfortunately, in sleep medicine, we have been dealing with the use of two scoring rules for identifying a type of respiratory event called a hypopnea. The rules for this are 4% or 3%. Medicare, among other payers, have adopted the 4% rule for scoring these events. It is important to keep in mind that while the 3% versus 4% may sound insignificant I can assure it is not. In many cases it has made the difference between patients receiving treatment or not.

There are three types of respiratory events we evaluate or score within the context of sleep testing. These events are—apnea, hypopnea, and respiratory effort-related arousal (typically only scored in presence of EEG-coupled recordings—PSG or HSAT (w/EEG component). The first two categories—apnea and hypopnea—can be further broken down into other classes *(see my previous article in Renegade Health Magazine Issue 1, Spring 2023)*.

Sleep apnea severity ultimately determines treatment options with the more severe apnea having less options overall. The severity scale for sleep apnea uses AHI or REI. RDI is NOT included for a sleep apnea diagnosis because the RDI is directly related to events that are not apnea. This doesn't mean that the RDI is not important. Quite the contrary, the RDI is incredibly important especially in symptomatic patients where the AHI or REI is normal.

This second article in the sleep series has taken us on a journey from common reporting terms and a breakdown of some of the data elements that we will see in a report. The next article is going to focus on the different treatment options that are available and how combination of therapies work as well. Don't miss future issues!

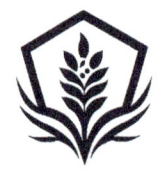

BowTied Hermit Crab *holds multiple certifications and accolades in the sleep world. He continues to be a student, teacher, and clinician in the field of sleep medicine for nearly 20 years. A believer in personalized patient-centered, accessible, high quality care with reasonable costs while improving outcomes.*

Want to be sure you are asking your sleep provider the right questions or have questions about this article? Contact him for a personalized review of your sleep data.

You can follow him on Twitter at:
@BTHermitCrab

And email him at:
bthermitcrab@pm.me

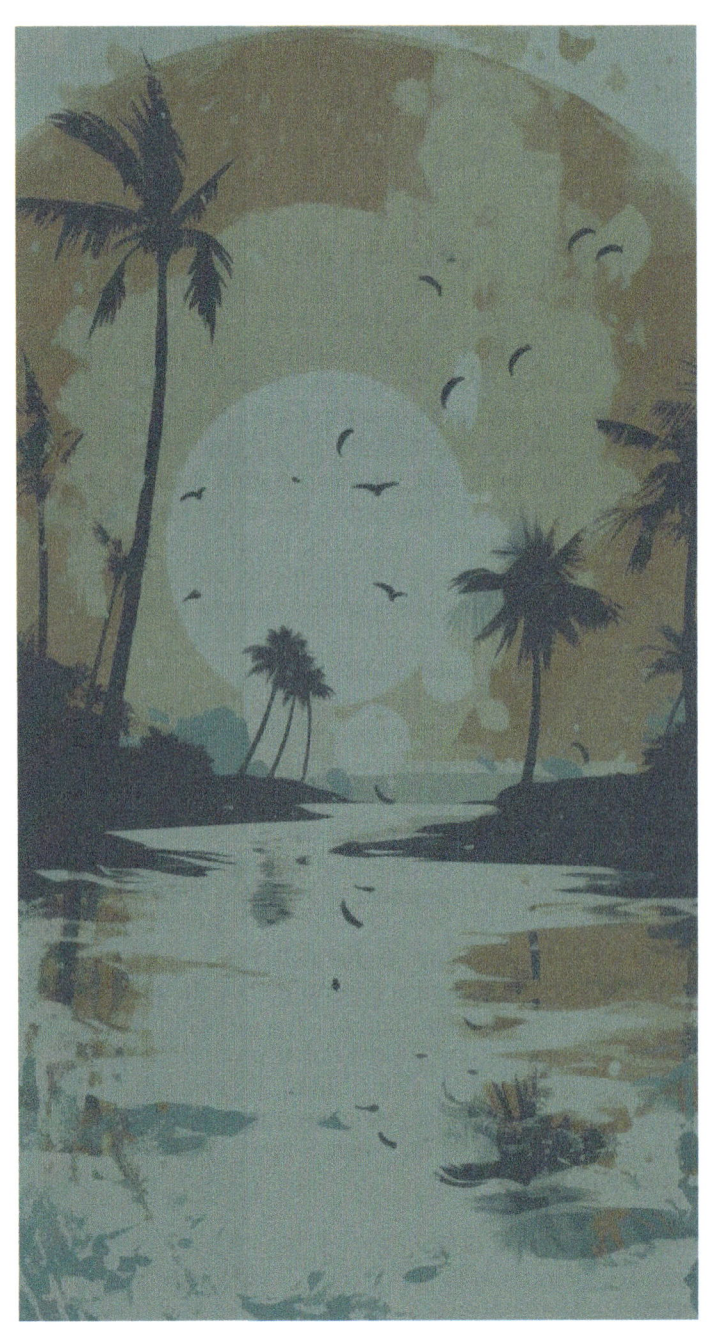

Warning: The "Red Pill" is True (sort of)

Leila Tomasone

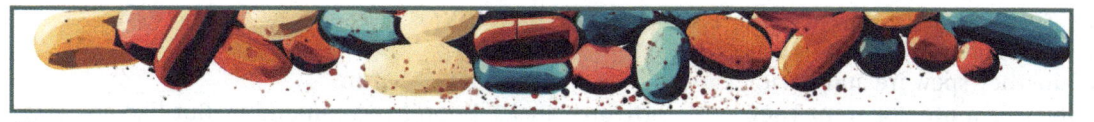

THE problem with the red pill is that it's right. Sort of.

And that's what makes it dangerous.

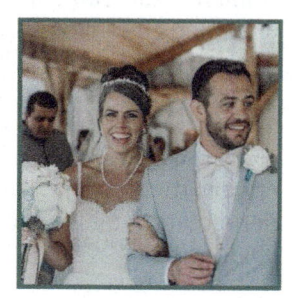

The Red Pill is an often-misunderstood concept that originated in the Men's Rights Movement. Men's rights bloggers (collectively called the "Manosphere") intended to empower men who felt powerless in their relationships with women. Men and women have very different needs in relationships, so content meant for men can offend women (and vice versa). Consequently, women who encounter and absorb red pill content can feel punched in the gut when they take it personally.

I first encountered red pill philosophy as a single mom over 35. I was proud of being a smart and logical person, but reacted emotionally to its messages. Red pill content focuses on bleak statistics about divorce, family courts, declining female fertility, and single motherhood, so I felt attacked. Ultimately, the facts forced me to grow. But then I had to move past the bleakness and find hope for my daughters and myself.[1]

I achieved that goal. I attracted and married a strong, protective man. For joy! My success compels me to share the possibilities and strategies for a positive outcome with other women. That's why I teach and coach women to date for marriage (if that's what they want), no matter their circumstances.

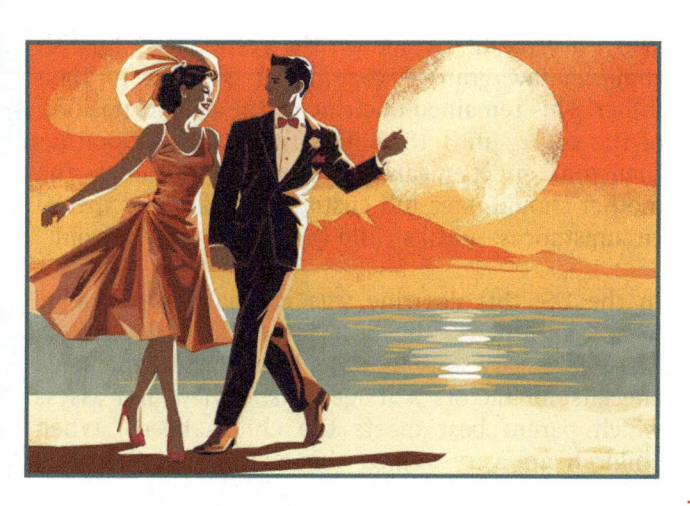

What is "The Red Pill"?

The concept of the red pill references the movie, The Matrix. It's based on the idea that, once one is exposed to reality in such a harsh light, there is no going back. The "blue pill" maintains the façade of the matrix—a false reality—where men remain unaware of women's true needs in relationships. Unawareness disadvantages men (and women) in relationships with the opposite sex. They believe niceness and household chores turn women on and make them stay committed. Statistics like "women initiate 70% of divorces" and anecdotes of men being "divorce raped" without any warning seem to prove the opposite.

Chris Williamson recently explained unconscious drives as "ultimate reasons" for our behavior. Ultimate reasons, in contrast to proximate reasons, are physiologic and evolutionary drivers that cause us to pursue behaviors that improve our chances of survival as an individual or as a species. There are also dysfunctional drivers for behavior that make sense given the environment we grew up in, but no longer serve us in the pursuit of healthy relationships. All these unconscious factors play into why we do what we do, even when we think our motives for taking our chosen actions are completely different. Such is true of men AND women.

> *Natural selection favours certain behaviours but doesn't necessarily favour us having explicit awareness of why we do what we do.*
>
> *Dr. Tania Reynolds*

Men are motivated by sex and other needs like responsibility and companionship... and that's a good thing! Women are motivated by commitment, romance, resource provision, procreation... and that's good, too! The proximate reason for our behaviors is that they feel good, but ultimately, there are deeper reasons.

Red pill men seem to epitomize the old cliché about women: "You can't live with 'em, and you can't live without 'em." Some go so far as to swear off relationships completely (also called MGTOW – Men Going Their Own Way). While they spew ire and vitriol against women on the daily, it is quite apparent they crave the company of a lovely lady. Unfortunately, they create their own self-fulfilling philosophy: they perpetuate the loneliness that made them unhappy to begin with.

Let's examine some common red pill tropes, and how you can look at them differently.

The Wall and the Empty Egg Carton
Red pillers talk a lot about women hitting "the wall" at a certain age, around 25. They claim this is when her looks and fertility drop, thus losing some of the power she used to have over desirable men. When she hits the wall, she then shifts her focus from short-term sexual relationships with powerful "Alphas" (referred to with vulgar slang terms) to long-term marriage and family with a "Beta" provider. *

Women have a biological clock. I hope this isn't news to anyone. (Men have one too, by the way.) So, the reality is, time does tend to take its toll on physical appearance. Physical appearance is mostly a function of health; the two tend to be closely related. Things become less elastic and shift around, bad habits start to catch up with us, and it isn't as easy to maintain good health and hot looks. In this way, The Red Pill has a point. Women can't have babies into old age.

Zoom in, and there's more to the story.

Men these days are less fertile than they used to be, too. People are getting married later and delaying their first child even further. Couples everywhere are coming to terms with infertility. They face a future without the families they desired, consciously or unconsciously.

Culture has changed our notions of marriage, and individuals are paying the price. Young men and women are both told to put off family goals in favor of career aspirations and financial "stability." In the past, those were pursuits for couples to tackle as a team. First, you get married and have babies. Then you start amassing some wealth and focus on your own personal fulfillment. That gave husbands and wives an opportunity to bond over shared desires, prior to gazing at each other and wondering, "what do you do to make me happy?" Nowadays, we're all chasing happiness and self-fulfillment, at the expense of family creation and true contentment.

Remember when you choose which lens through which to view the opposite sex, we've all absorbed harmful cultural messages that could account for delays in maturity?

"Never date a single mom"
Divorce sucks. I don't recommend it! But like any test or trial, it can also teach some very valuable lessons. I learned a lot and changed a lot because of my first, dysfunctional marriage and divorce. But learning and changing are not automatic. Real change takes a lot of discipline. Someone who has made the easy but wrong choices will tend to do so in the future too. In this way, the red pill position is truthful.

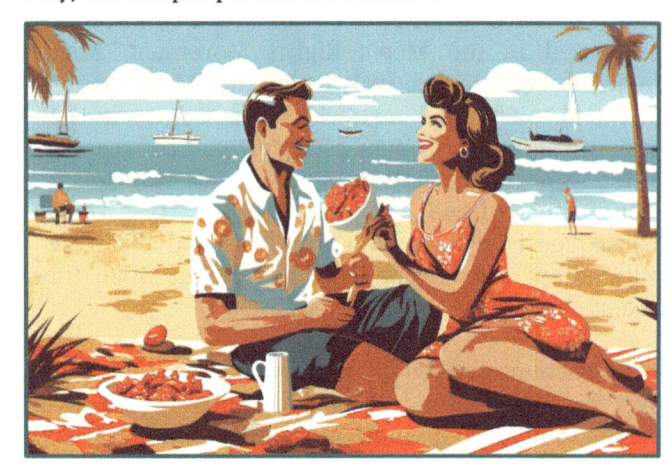

It isn't often that people truly change, but it does happen. *The key is to ask the right questions and judge the evidence as objectively as possible.* Love and attraction are blinding for most people. Sometimes we assume mistakenly that we can help, rescue, or fix someone (nice guy behavior, also called white knighting) who has made mistakes or had bad things happen to them in their past. This is a dangerous temptation that prevents real, sustainable love and commitment. *Consider the impulse to rescue your partner a big red flag.*

When divorce first came on the scene, early English common law granted custody of children to their father. This remained doctrine as the default position of the courts until 1873. The Tender Years Doctrine then took effect, meaning that courts presumed the mother should have full custody—barring any special circumstances—until a child was at least 16 years old.

In the US, this doctrine was gradually replaced by what's known as "the best interests of the child." These laws vary state by state, but generally there is a checklist of factors a judge must review and assess which parent best meets the child's needs. When children are very young, this may mean the main caregiver would be given primary custody. The other parent would then be given some schedule of evening and weekend visitation.

The best interests of the child change as the child gets older, and courts are granting joint custody more often. Joint custody requires communication and cooperation between the parents, however, and that can be a difficulty in contested custody.

Most custody decisions (80-90%) are made without going to court. The 10-20% that aren't decided out of court are by definition "high conflict" and tend to involve one or more parties with cluster B personality disorders – BPD or NPD. It is almost impossible to coparent with one of those personalities, so the most contentious cases aren't good candidates for joint custody. These are the cases where false accusations and parental alienation run rampant.

That's why we need to avoid it if possible. But that doesn't make opting out the only or even the best plan. The key is to choose your spouse carefully AND go into marriage with the right perspective. It's not divorce that ruins men, it's picking the wrong partner and not knowing how to maintain a healthy marriage.

"She's not yours, it's just your turn"

Successful, "alpha" men know the benefits of a good woman by your side, building your family, committing to stay married, and maintaining "frame" that ensures a mutually satisfying relationship.

86% of millionaires are married. Rich, powerful men understand the value of marriage. Men who would rather never have a penny to their name than ever risk paying alimony and child support often do just that: they never accumulate any meaningful wealth and never have anything at risk! Meanwhile, men with the most to risk usually have stable marriages. Why is that? Maybe they know something you don't know.

If you aspire to be successful, pay attention to what the best and most successful people are doing. Start with a strong marriage. According to Entrepreneur.com, "Being married helps you earn more money... The statistics are clear: Marriage and income are strongly correlated. According to the research, one of the biggest reasons why married people are more productive and make money is because they have a partner pushing them."

But, "he's the prize!"

Red pillers claim that "he's the prize" in the relationship, not her, and that this is the correct lens with which to view male/female dynamics. But is that true? Ideally, both partners should believe they have the better end of the deal!

However, research has shown that stronger and longer-lasting marriages tend to involve husbands who are head-over-heels for their wives. The Bible instructs, "...rejoice in the wife of your youth...let her breasts fill you at all times with delight; be intoxicated always in her love" (Prov. 5:18-23). Choose your love, and then love your choice! A wife should be her husband's standard of beauty.

This is the kind of dynamic I teach my clients to pursue. This is what brings women the greatest sense of security, which is what we need to feel satisfied and settled in our relationship. Security allows a woman to relax into her feminine to the degree necessary for rearing children.

For women, being left when pregnant or with young children is our worst nightmare. And on the flip side, the ability to relax is an essential aspect of feminine behavior, pregnancy, birth, breastfeeding, and child rearing. An anxious and insecure woman is not a woman most men want to be around! Pregnancy and the postpartum period can intensely exacerbate depression and anxiety, so you certainly do not want to come into a marriage or parenthood with that as the default state.

The statistical research quoted in this tweet further reinforces that "she's the prize" relationships may indeed have an advantage over "he's the prize" relationships. When women believe their husband is the better catch, they also tend to believe that he will cheat on them, making them more likely to cheat preemptively. Crazy stuff! The point: you can probably find statistics to support whatever perspective you want to believe. So why not believe what is more constructive and gives you the best opportunity at a happy, healthy, and successful relationship?

You Can't Negotiate Desire!

Red pill men tend to obsess over women's desire. Obsessing over what our partner wants or doesn't want and what they think about us is an easy cycle to get sucked into: it's called codependency. That inevitably brings about more of what we DON'T want in the relationship. The better approach is to focus on our own path to success and happiness, which ultimately makes us so much more attractive and desirable! Make an inventory of what you want to achieve:

- Career
- Hobbies
- Friends
- Fitness

How is your progress? Are there some goals you've been neglecting or not admitting to yourself? Often when we feel dissatisfied with our own abilities or achievements, our partner's flaws, shortcomings, criticisms, or wrong opinions are just too tempting to ignore.

What are your relationship goals? Do you aspire to be in a connected and romantic relationship? What can you do to bolster your side of the equation? Re-focusing on our own role is a sure-fire path to increased satisfaction and can cause a surge of confidence, attraction, and passion. Any number of positive side effects!

Conclusion

The manosphere makes some great points, but when the complaints become an excuse to stay stuck, we need to choose a different perspective. While the Red Pill offers a certain degree of truth, it can also lead to negative thinking patterns that prevent people from having healthy relationships and marriages. To help you avoid getting stuck in this way of thinking, I want to give you some reframes and strategies so you can have better-functioning relationships:

⇒ Choose a different perspective. Notice how negative statistics may be accurate in broad, general terms; but on an individual level, the meaning is often lost or incorrect. Mindset gives us the option to choose our perspective. Focus on the positive to improve your odds of success and happiness.

⇒ Acknowledge and respect sex differences in relationship objectives. Self-interest is an important ingredient in strong relationships. Men and women need different things, and it's healthy to pursue those opposing goals. The complementary energies, desires, and talents of men and women create and hold the beautiful tension that bonds us together and sustains the species.

⇒ Refocus on your own goals. If you feel yourself getting sucked into negativity and complaining about the opposite sex, remind yourself of what you want to achieve. Making forward progress will make you more attractive and help you have a healthy relationship in the future.

⇒ Follow what successful people do to be successful yourself. There are plenty of happy couples out there. Find some who have what you want in life, and study what they do to get what they have.

⇒ Date intentionally and only accept respectful treatment. Marriage is good for people who do it consciously and develop themselves, but it has disastrous consequences for those who fall into it haphazardly. You teach people how to treat you, as they say. Only continue relationships that are supportive and encouraging.

* These definitions aren't accurate statistically; I'm just relating the red pill perspective here.

Notes:

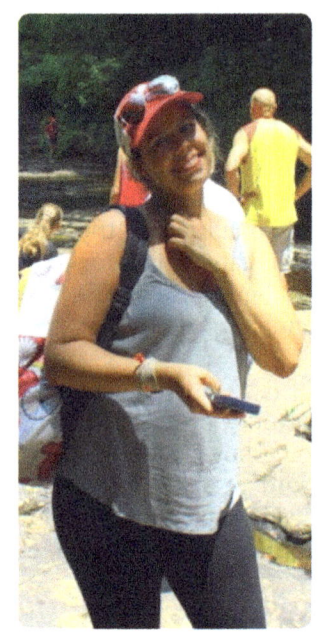

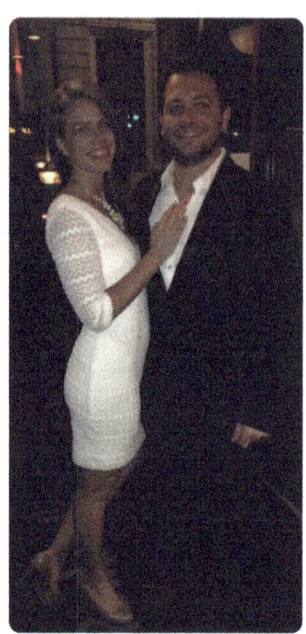

1. The left image is me in 2014, and the image on the right is me in 2017 (age 36 vs. age 39), with my now-husband. Sometimes the clock rewinds!

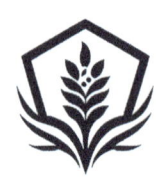

Leila Tomasone *helps women date in the 21st century, and manifest a healthy & lasting marriage. She focuses on masculine-feminine dynamics, mindset, & high value feminine abundance.*

You can follow her on Twitter at:
@LimitlessLeila

And see her Website at:
https://leilatomasone.com

Meet Your Protein Demands

Harsh Strongman

> **WHEN** I started lifting, I knew eating lots of protein was important, but I could not figure out how to get enough protein on a vegetarian diet. I read all the articles on the topic and found them to be nonsensical and unhelpful. Over the years, I've figured out what works and what doesn't. I can say that most of the information found online is garbage.

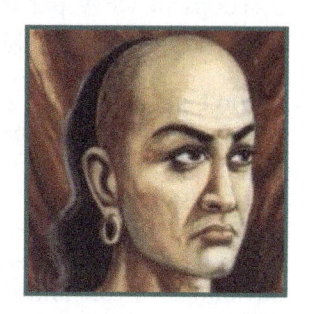

Most articles on "How to get more protein for vegetarians" are written by people with zero practical experience.

I read all the articles about high protein vegetarian Indian diets online back in the day, and even today, I find that most articles on the topic are written by journalism interns and people who have no idea what they're talking about.

For example, most articles on how to get more protein as a vegetarian say "eat mung sprouts". It's often their #1 recommendation. And it's utterly ridiculous.

While it's true that mung sprouts are protein-rich (they've got a decent amount of protein on a per-calorie basis), there's just no way that you can eat enough of them to get a decent amount of protein in you.

Let's say you eat 400 grams of mung sprouts. That's a LOT of mung sprouts. It'll make a hefty lunch for many people.

And how much protein did you get for your entire meal?

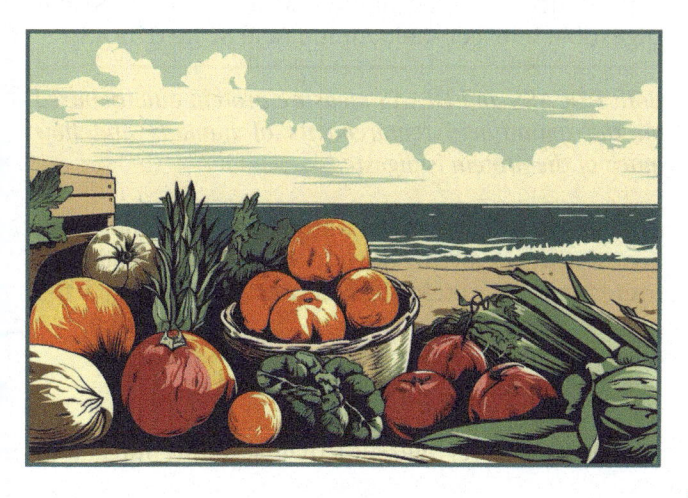

Only 16 grams.

In other words, there's no way you can get a decent amount of protein eating tons of mung sprouts, despite the fact that mung sprouts are "rich in protein".

The same applies to a lot of other foods that are recommended in these articles: pulses, legumes, dals, etc. While it's true that they are protein-rich, there's no way you can eat them in the large quantities you'd need to get the amount of protein you require as someone whose strength training.

I've even read articles that recommend eating soy. This is horrible advice. Soy is terrible for a man's hormonal balance because it contains plant-based estrogens. If you are a man, you should avoid processed soy as much as possible.

Most articles on getting more protein for vegetarians are written by people with zero practical experience. They are written by people who don't lift but went to school and learned that "soy, dals, legumes and sprouts are high in protein" in science class. They are just regurgitating the same things in their articles with different words.

[Note: This is not to demonize mung beans. Mung is rich in micronutrients and should absolutely be consumed. However, if they form your primary source of protein, you're living in a make-believe academic world.]

Before I get into the actual meat of the article – I want to address two things:

1. How much protein do you need in a day?
2. Does the source of protein matter (i.e. is the protein from milk as good as the protein from dal, and if not, then which is better?)

There are a lot of bad articles about this topic as well, but for different reasons. I've seen estimates as high as 2 grams per *pound* of body weight, but they're all mostly written by companies trying to sell you lots of protein powder. If you listen to them, you'd be eating 5 scoops of whey per day and still struggle to meet their *minimum* protein goals.

I won't get too much into this, but if you want the science and studies behind it, read the article at (https://mennohenselmans.com/the-myth-of-1glb-optimal-protein-intake-for-bodybuilders/).

Here is the short version: There is normally no advantage to consuming more than 0.82g/lb (1.8g/kg) of protein per day to preserve or build muscle for *natural trainees*. This already includes a mark-up, since most research finds no more benefits after 0.64g/lb (1.4g/kg).

Further, this assumes that you're lean. If you're obese, you'd need to deduct the body fat % from your weight to find out your lean body mass and use that as a metric to calculate how much protein you need to eat.

For example, if you're 120 kg and are at 40% body fat, you'd need to use 120*(1-0.4) = 72 kg as your lean body mass metric.

To calculate your body fat percentage, all you need is a pair of skin fold fat calipers.

Enter your skin fold measurements into any online calculator and it should give you a pretty good estimate.

If you are strength training, you should aim to get at least 1.4 grams of protein per kg of lean body mass and ideally try to get 1.8 grams per kg.

You can eat more protein if you like–it's healthy and is the most thermogenic of the three macronutrients–there are no disadvantages to eating more protein. However, if you're reading this article, you're probably struggling to hit your 1.4-1.8 grams a day, and not worrying about overshooting.

Most vegetarian Indians eat about 40–50 grams of protein in a day, which is really low. Other than a lack of exercise, this is one of the reasons why most Indian youths are physically weak (almost always either obese or skinny fat) – they just don't get enough protein in.

If you want to be strong, you need to eat enough protein. Your muscles are made up of protein and if you're not eating enough protein you won't have enough muscle and you won't be strong.

Is All Protein The Same?
No. And for two reasons: 1) Digestibility and 2) Amino-Acid Profile.

Protein Digestibility
Not all foods are digested equally by humans. Some food sources have a lot of their protein end up in our feces while protein from other food sources gets completely absorbed.

Amino Acid Profile
Protein is composed of amino-acids. Different protein sources have different amino-acid profiles. There are 9 essential amino-acids, where the word essential means that the mammal body cannot synthesize them and we must get them from our diets.

In general, plant based sources of protein tend to be deficient in one or more essential amino acids. If you get most of your protein from plants – you have to get your protein from a variety of plant sources so you can get all the essential amino-acids in adequate quantities.

Animal based protein sources tend to be rich in all amino-acids needed to build muscle. This is simply because when you eat protein from an animal, the animal has already done the work of eating different plants and turning the plant protein into protein they can store in the form of muscle.

Obviously, animal muscle has all the amino acids you need to create muscle in your own body, as you are also an animal.

This is not normally too much of a problem as most Indian vegetarians usually consume a variety plant sources of protein (like grains with dals), but it's worth knowing.

Putting The Two Together
There are two measures for how much protein a food actually provides to the human body – Protein digestibility-corrected amino acid score (PDCAAS) and Digestible Indispensable Amino Acid Score (DIAAS).

Both PDCASS and DIAAS measure protein quality based on the amino-acid requirements of humans and how much of the protein is digested.

PDCAAS is an older measure that considers the entire digestive tract all the way to fecal matter and thus overestimates protein digestion as it also counts the protein absorbed by bacteria in the large intestine.

PDCAAS is less accurate than DIAAS.

DIAAS is a newer measure that accounts for amino

acid digestibility until the end of the small intestine.

DIAAS is a more accurate measure of amino acids absorbed by the body and the protein's contribution to human amino acid and nitrogen requirements.

At the right is a chart showing different foods along with their PDCAAS and DIAAS scores:

As you can see, animal protein sources tend to be superior in quality to plant protein sources both in terms of amino-acids and digestibility.

This is not me demonizing plant protein, but it's simply a result of the fact that when you eat animal proteins (milk, eggs, meat, etc.) – the animal has already done the hard work of turning the protein from plants into protein suitable for animals (in composition and form).

NOTE: This article is an adapted excerpt from the article "How To Increase Protein In Indian Vegetarian Diet (With Desi Diet Plan)." You can read the full article at:
https://lifemathmoney.com/how-to-increase-protein-in-indian-vegetarian-diet-with-desi-diet-plan/

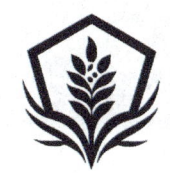

Harsh Strongman *is better known on Twitter as LifeMathMoney.*

You can follow him on Twitter at:
@LifeMathMoney

And read his newsletter at:
https://newsletter.lifemathmoney.com

DIAAS and PDCAAS Scores of various food sources.

	PDCAAS	DIAAS
Milk Protein Concentrate	1	1.18
Pork		1.17
Whole Milk Powder	1	1.159
Whole Milk	1	1.14
Egg (Hard Boiled)	1	1.13
Whey Protein Isolate	1	1.09
Chicken Breast	1	1.08
Egg		1.01
Potato	0.99	1
Soybean	1	0.996
Chickpeas	0.74	0.83
Pea Protein Concentrate	0.893	0.822
Peas	0.782	0.647
Cooked Rice	0.616	0.595
Cooked Kidney Beans	0.648	0.588
Oats		0.57
Tofu	0.56	0.52
Roasted Peanuts	0.509	0.434
Wheat	0.463	0.40-0.48
Almonds	0.39	0.4
Corn	0.37	0.36
Legumes	0.70-0.89	0.68-0.88

ISSUE 2 SUMMER 2023

Take Control of Your Food Chain

BowTied Farmer

> **THE** year is 2035. You wake up to start your day. Head to the refrigerator to grab your bottle of cockroach milk and pour some into your K-Pod cup of coffee that is really just... more cockroaches. For breakfast you stop to have a bagel from Stardonald's on the way to work riding on your government mandated electric scooter.

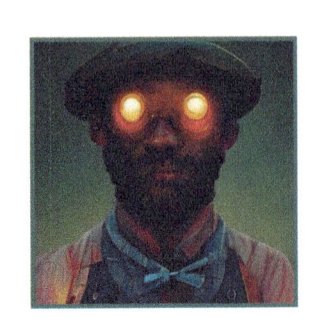

Meat and eggs are no longer available in the US ever since the Green New Deal 33.0 was enacted by Emperor AOC.

You are required to commute to work this year since you were found to be posting negative comments about your local mayor on Twittbok. When you arrive home that night your groceries for the week have been delivered. No meat, no dairy, no eggs, no produce. Everything is in shiny plastic wrappers filled with highly processed food using the latest GMO laboratories.

Foods that were once made with seed oils are now made with bugs from the WEF conglomerates that started popping up back in 2022. You are also on several medications that have been mandated to ensure you are a productive member of society.

Then you wake up. What a terrible nightmare!

However, this nightmare can become reality. It's time we fought back against Big Food and Big Government by taking control of our food chain. How? I'm glad you asked!

Take Control of Your Food Chain

In grade school we learned about the food chain, it was a sequence in ecology that transferred matter and energy in the form of food from organism to organism.

There is a food chain for humans and it has changed rapidly in recent decades. Today, most people don't even think about where the food they are eating comes from. Many don't realize that most food on the grocery store shelves is still grown by a farmer.

In the old days, almost everyone was a farmer.

The industrial revolution brought about massive change where people could make money by working for someone else in a factory. With more and more people at work in a factory, they weren't able to grow their own food and raise their animals. This is where the idea of massive farming and food supply shifted from small and local to big and corporate.

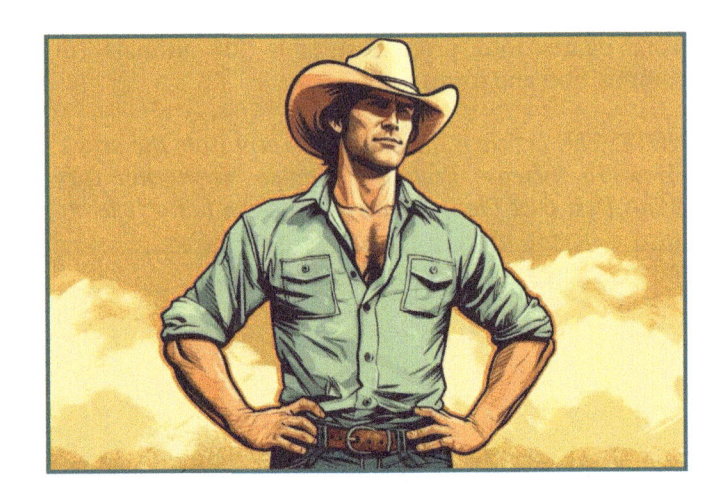

Along with this new food supply chain system, the global market was opened which allows us to eat fresh bananas in the dead of winter. We are also blessed with the luxury of being able to drive our vehicles to a place called Costco and pick up giant bags of frozen blueberries, strawberries, and just about any type of food you could ever want.

In a perfect world, this system is the best because it allows us to get access to a wide variety of fresh(er) food year round. It allows farmers to focus on growing crops and animals that thrive in their location. In a global market, this is the most efficient way. However, with all the advancement in production with our new global food supply chain, there have been many compromises, cost increases, and negative effects on our environment. Surprise!

Nowadays, it doesn't make sense for a family to stay home and grow all the food they need for the entire year. If everyone had to grow their own food, many people would not be able to enjoy fruits and crops that aren't available in their location due to climate or soil conditions.

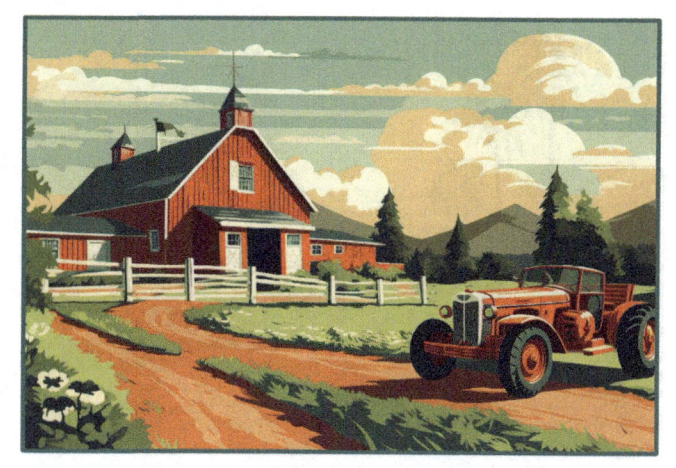

The food chain we have today works because it's easy for consumers and profitable for large corporations. Nobody has time to grow their own food anymore, and even if they did, most people wouldn't because... well... it's hard. The amount of work it takes to grow edible food from a seed or harvest beef from a cow is daunting, startup and operating costs are high, and regulations are thick.

It's obvious why most people today aren't growing their own food for their families anymore. You may not be able to grow your own food, but you can at least start sourcing your food from local farmers. There are several reasons why you should start looking for local sources of food, I'll cover most of them here.

Rising Food Costs at the Grocery Stores

Unless you've been living in an off grid cabin in the upper peninsula eating MRE's for the past three years, you've noticed the price of food at the grocery stores, high!

Here is the CPI data for the costs of food since 2020.[1]

- Eggs 40%
- Poultry 25%
- Fats and Oils 24%
- Beef and Pork 23%
- Dairy 20%
- Fresh Fruit and Vegetables 11.6%

There are many factors that have led to the increase in the price of food. Some may say that it's by design. Government policies in the wake of Covid-19 have definitely caused prices to increase due to massive money printing, lockdowns, and giving people money to stay home instead of going to work. The war in Ukraine and other foreign policies haven't helped.

Startup costs for farming operations are higher than ever. The cost to fence an acre of land for raising cows is anywhere from $10k-$27k. The cost of animal feed has risen almost 30% in the last 3 years. Everything required to set up a food processing or growing operation has pretty much doubled in cost. Diesel fuel costs have risen causing the transportation of food to cost more than it used to.

Adding fuel to the fire is large food processing companies are putting the squeeze on farmers and ranchers offering low prices for bulk produce and meat because of the decrease in the amount of food processing plants across the country. You can read more about the meat packing companies in a great article by BowTied Rancher.[2]

Finding food from a local source (a Farmer) allows you and the producer to cut out the middleman. Which will not only reduce your cost, it will support someone who is out there every day trying to make a difference by producing food. The small farmers are struggling right now due to the reasons I just listed. If you find a good local farmer that you can trust, support them (with money).

Chemical Free Food

Another great reason to find a local source of food is trust. A good friend on Twitter wrote a great thread on this topic as I was writing this article.[3]

Since you are reading this article right now, I assume that you are tuned into the amount of chemicals and pesticides that our food chain has been compromised with. Finding food that is clean from pesticides and GMO products is a tall task in today's world.

If you're like me, you question everything. You may have asked yourself, is this apple really organic? Sure, it says it on the sticker, but how do you know?

To be honest, we really don't know. The only way to truly know is to know the farmer who is producing the food. I'll show you how.

Most fruits, vegetables, and other food items are imported from foreign countries where regulations are much more lax or even non-existent. Sure, there are USDA standards for organic operations that export food into our country.[4] But do you really trust the USDA to monitor farming operations in Central America? In my opinion, the farther you get from the source of your food, the farther you are from a trustworthy source.

Not only do you want to find food that is not riddled with pesticides, you also need to know how foreign countries fertilize their crops. In places like Mexico, farmers have been using raw sewage straight from Mexico City to irrigate and fertilize their crops. Many vegetables that you eat on your dinner table from the grocery store could be coming from a farm like this.[5] You might be thinking "Yeah, but that only happens in Third World countries right?" Wrong, a farm in Michigan was caught using untreated human waste for fertilization of their produce just last year.[6]

Unsustainably Grown Meat and Produce
The last big reason it's important to source your food locally from a small farmer is sustainability. Large agricultural operations for meat and produce are getting more and more unsustainable. There's not much you can do about this problem because to be quite honest, without our current agricultural processes, many people would go hungry.

The cold hard truth is our current agricultural system is extremely efficient. The use of pesticides has revolutionized agriculture. Advancements in the cattle industry have allowed us to almost double the amount of beef harvested from a single steer.

The problem? It's unsustainable. It's causing problems with our environment and our health. While it's easy to simply choose organic labels at the grocery store, these products are still coming from massive growing operations that are causing problems for our environment. If you really care about the environment, you would find a local grower and support them. Their carbon footprint is a tiny fraction of the one General Mills is making. Tread lightly.

I know it's easy (and cheaper) to go to the big stores and stock up on everything you need for the week in one trip. That's fine, but I'm pushing you to find a few small farmers to get maybe one or two staples from instead. By doing this, you're supporting a real person you can talk to and shake hands with. You know where it is coming from, and you know it's fresh. It's important to build relationships like this in a time when these small farmers are actively being pushed out of the market by Big Corporations.

Not to mention the feeling when you're eating fresh eggs and milk from your Farmer Friend, when the grocery store is completely out due to some new disease or issue with the food chain.

How to Find a Local Farmer
I'll tell you how I found several local sources of food and made many friends in the process.

To start, you want to be looking for someone who can supply you with your everyday staples so that you can easily buy from them weekly. Items like milk, eggs, produce, fruit, and meat. You're probably not going to find someone locally growing exotic fruits or high-end beef. You'll still be using Costco or the grocery store, we're just looking for the basics.

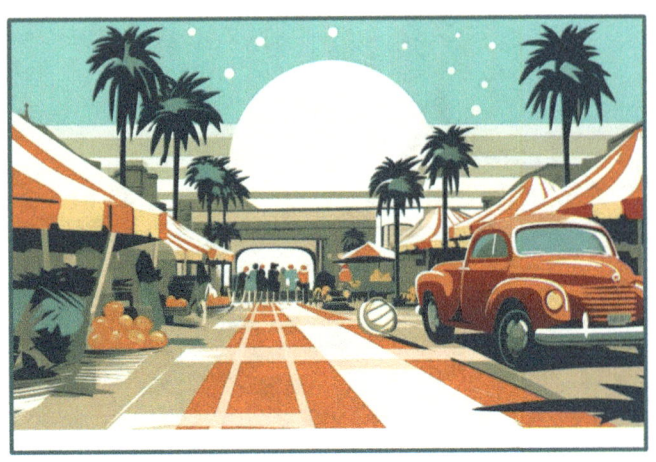

Finding a Farmer at the Farmers Market
When people think about finding locally grown food, they think about a Farmer's Market. While this can be a successful journey, it's important to know that not all sellers at the Farmer's Market are actually producing that product. Many of the sellers at farmers markets and produce stands in small towns are just resellers. They buy produce in bulk and resell it. It's usually coming from the same places the grocery stores are getting their produce. In many cases it's not organic and the person selling it doesn't even know where it came from!

If you go to the Farmer's Market, you want to be looking for a farmer to make friends with. Someone who will talk to you and tell you about their operation. You want to find the man with dirty hands. You should be looking to build a relationship, not just cross out an item on your grocery list.

Ask them questions like:

- Where do you grow these items?
- How long have you been farming?
- Do you use any pesticides on your crops?
- I'm very interested in local farmers. Can I visit your farm one day?

These questions will quickly give you an idea if this is someone you would like to begin supporting with your hard-earned cash. You're looking for someone that operates fairly close to where you live. If they say they would allow you to visit their farm, take them up on it! There's nothing better than driving out to a small farm and seeing how some of their day-to-day works. My wife and I have made this one of our favorite "dates".

If you find someone who fits the bill and is growing something you're interested in, congrats! Great success! After you begin to purchase from your new farmer friend, you can ask them where they get their milk, eggs, and meat. They probably know someone who grows the other items on your list.

However, this may not work for you. Many good small farmers have stopped going to the Farmer's Market because it's just not a smart economical decision for them. They're getting hammered right now due to the many costs listed earlier. Some of them are even having to take day jobs to support their small farm operations due to the rising costs. The customers are going to Costco on Saturday, not Farmer's Markets. Why would a small farmer spend a whole Saturday at a Farmer's Market where the crowd is dwindling and not make very many sales? They have more important work to do.

Finding a Farmer on Social Media

Today's small farmer's are primarily using Facebook and Instagram for marketing and networking. I've found more Chad Farmers in my area on Facebook than any other. The process is similar to the Farmer's Market, except it's all on social media.

Here are the steps for finding a Local Farmer on Facebook:

1. Go on Facebook and find the Groups Section.
2. Search for groups like "Cattle Farmers of Central Florida" or "Backyard Chickens of Central Florida" or "Organic Gardening in Central Florida", etc.
3. Many groups will pop up, you want to make sure you're joining the ones with the most members, and it will tell you how frequent and how many posts are happening. You want to find the most active groups.
4. Join these groups and begin to check your feed, you'll start to see posts from small farm pages that are shared into the group.

Be on the lookout for whatever you're looking for. If you see someone post a beautiful garden offering fresh produce, you might have a winner! Looking for fresh food can also be as simple as asking the group. In the gardening group ask something like "I'm looking for a local organic veggie share in Ocala, Florida." or in the cattle farmers group, ask something like "I'm looking to purchase half of beef in Ocala, Florida".

Depending on your location, you should get several suggestions. Go down the list looking at the people that were suggested. See if you can find their farm page or website, from there you can see if they look like someone you could trust. Try to get an idea of the the size of their operation and maybe even find some reviews. When you talk to them make sure you remember that you're trying to build a relationship, not just fill your freezer. See if you can meet them and see their operation. You may even be able to pick out your cow!!

Here are some general precautions to use when picking your new local farm source of food:

For meat producers, it's very important to try to find customer reviews. Buying meat direct from a farmer is expensive and you're getting a large amount of meat at one time. You need to be sure you're going to get quality meat that tastes good. Don't rush the meat farmer search! Once you find a reputable cattle farmer, you'll work out the details. Usually you pay the farmer and he takes the live cattle to the butcher. You pick the meat up from the butcher. Most butcher facilities for cattle are required to be USDA certified, so you don't have to worry too much about the butchering facility. You just want to make sure the rancher knows what he's doing.

There are many factors that go into the quality and taste of meat. How the animal was raised, what it was fed, when it was fed in the days leading up to the butcher. Do your own research and make sure you're getting what you want.

For other items like raw milk, it's very important to see their operation. You want to make sure the area where the milk is poured into jars is clean. Make sure they have the proper equipment to process the milk safely like clean glass jars and clean equipment. Milk should be iced down shortly after it is harvested so you will want to see an ice machine somewhere on the property. General food safe practices should be in place when the milk is being handled.

Veggie and fruit operations are less intense. You're just looking for someone who doesn't use synthetic chemicals on their produce and that the food is actually being grown on the property.

Your egg source should be someone who cares for their chickens properly. Look for healthy looking birds that have plenty of room to walk. The chicken house is not going to be perfectly clean, but you want to try to make sure they're collecting eggs regularly and storing them properly. You'll know if you get a bad egg!!

Repeat this searching process until you're getting all of your main food staples from a trustworthy, local source regularly.

Summing It All Up

At the end of the day, we know our food chain is a total mess. The solution to all the big problems with our food chain is a small farmer.

Most people are trying to eat healthy by buying organic which is great. But most of the organic food suppliers are still mega corporations who don't care about you or your family. In order to make a difference, we must support local producers by building relationships with them and buying their goods regularly. Knowing where your food comes from is powerful. Small farmers are saving our planet by operating on a small scale. They take care of the land because they have too, it's their livelihood.

I hope you found this article helpful. If you would like to support me, please go to my website and try some of our products from my Farmer's Market store at https://bowtiedfarmer.com

Sources

1. https://www.ers.usda.gov/data-products/food-price-outlook/
2. https://bowtiedrancher.substack.com/p/lets-take-down-the-big-meat-packers
3. https://twitter.com/reallytanman/status/1654151134045433856
4. https://www.ams.usda.gov/services/organic-certification/international-trade/how-does-usda-assess-organic-equivalency-other-countries
5. https://www.foxnews.com/world/in-mexico-fears-a-new-plant-will-kill-wastewater-farming
6. https://www.mlive.com/news/ann-arbor/2022/10/produce-from-michigan-farm-using-untreated-human-waste-declared-public-health-risk.html

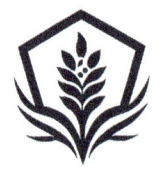

BowTied Farmer *is a father of three and Husband to an amazing mother and animal lover. Together they are striving to grow their own food and raise animals the way God intended. They homeschool their children and strive to live a healthy and fulfilling life, The Natural Life. They run a small apiary and make handcrafted goods which can be purchased at* https://bowtiedfarmer.com/

You can follow him on Twitter at:
@bowtiedfarmer

And read his Substack at:
https://bowtiedfarmer.substack.com

Personal Success Story

by Daniel
@clearly_caneda

I lost my mother to breast cancer at age 10 and I went from an active swimmer to someone who would struggle with weight for the next 32 years. I dabbled with weight lifting my senior year of high school and became fairly strong, but never maintained consistency.

Fast Forward to late January 2022, I was increasingly fearful of the consequences of a sedentary life and that set the groundwork for Michael of GainTrust to invite me to the Discord server. I joined, but I was just going to lose some weight and get stronger. That didn't last long.

The GainTrust community began to reframe my perception of health and fitness! Unfortunately, I came across my first obstacle when I messaged Mike stating I was going to have to take a long break to recoup from bicep tendonitis. It was then I decided to delete that message and tell Mike that I was not quitting and that though I was injured, I would still see success regardless. From that moment, I did nothing but cardio and leg exercises. Around May 2022 I lost my first nine pounds and my testosterone levels began to rise. As of today, I've lost 70 pounds.

The support I get from GainTrust has made all the difference in the world. The coaches have been there for me during the lowest points of my recovery, to my successes with weight loss. Now, I want more. With the help of GainTrust and the 100 Club, I have come to enjoy the gym and I look forward to sculpting the body that I want.

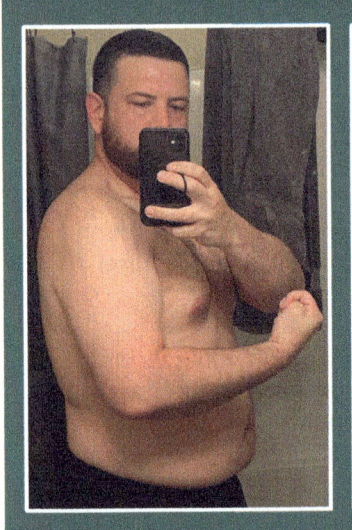

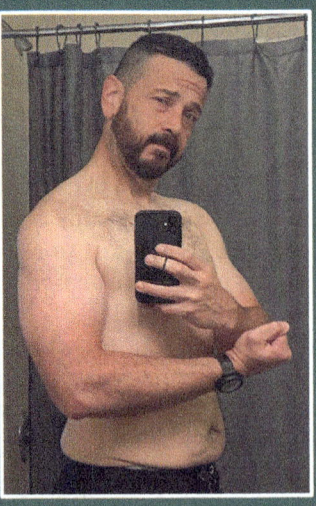

ISSUE 2   SUMMER 2023

Get Prepared for The Cold and Flu Season

BowTied Mrs Garden

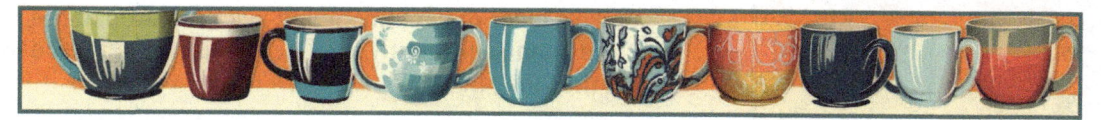

IF you're reading this, it's likely you're the type of person who holds themselves accountable for their health and wellness.

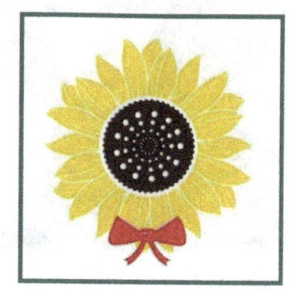

For those of us in the Northern hemisphere it's summer and you're probably making sure you're eating well, exercising, getting outside in the sun for vitamin D, and not really putting too much thought into cold and flu season which is only a few short months away.

If you want to make sure you and your family have access to some of the best virus busting herbal remedies, the time to make them is now! This ensures they are fully potent and ready for use before you need them. I'm here to offer a few basic recipes that you can make now and let marinate for the next couple months so that you have a fully prepared first line of defense come cold and flu season.

These are what I like to have ready and on hand before the first cases start showing up at school and work:

- Elderberry Syrup/Elixir Fire Cider
- Tea blends
- Fermented Garlic/Ginger Honey

These four remedies can help build your immunity so that in conjunction with healthy habits, diet and sanitation, you don't catch anything in the first place. But let's be real. We can do so much and still get sick.

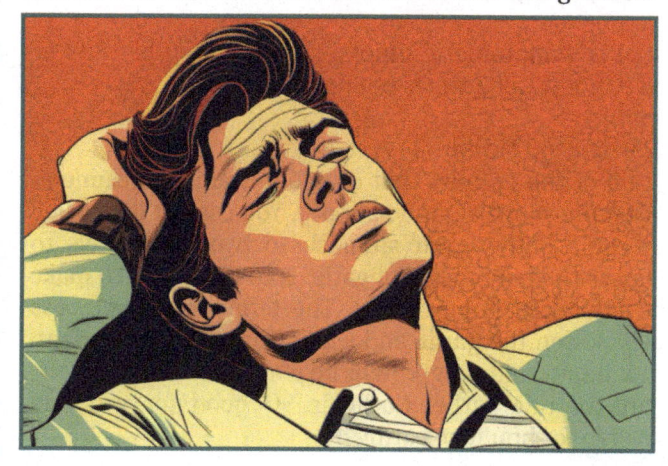

These remedies will also help your body fight nasty viruses so that you feel better, faster. As always, this is not medical advice! You should do your own research and seek out a trusted naturopath, doctor, or herbalist with any questions about your body and your health.

Elderberry Syrup/Elixir

Elderberry is my go-to for immunity—1 tbsp every day during cough and cold season. When symptoms start to manifest I go to 3 to 4 tbsp per day. Feel free to make this now and use it as a preventative. It will stay in your fridge for several weeks. You can also make your elixir and freeze it so that you can pop it out this fall when you may need it more. The following is a basic recipe but you can make as much as you want as long as you are consistent with your measurements!

- 2 Cups of dried elderberries
- 4 Cups Water (purified)
- Cinnamon Sticks (1-3)
- Ginger (dried or fresh to taste, 3 tsp dried is good)
- Clove to taste

Other Herbs if you like: ¼ of each Mullein, Astragalus, Rose Hips Raw Local Honey, or Raw Honey from a trusted source (see BowTiedFarmer's article in this issue for a link to purchase his Honey), Vodka or Brandy (if you don't want to freeze it)

Combine your berries, cinnamon, ginger and other herbs with the cold water in a pot and bring to a boil. Reduce heat and simmer for 40 minutes, covered. Remove from heat and steep for an additional hour. As they simmer, make sure to mash your berries a couple of times.

Carefully, as the concoction will still be pretty hot, strain the elderberry/herbals with a double cheesecloth and a funnel, and squeeze out all the liquid into a measurable container.

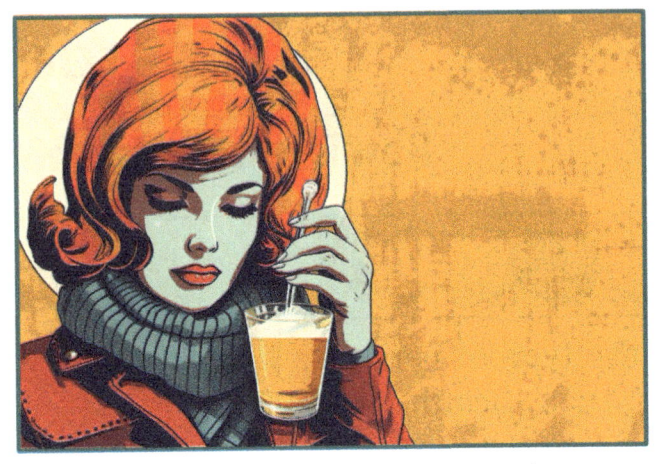

Allow the liquid to cool to just warmer than room temperature and add an equal amount of raw honey to the liquid. (1 cup of liquid, 1 cup of honey etc.)

At this point, you can choose to refrigerate or freeze. Refrigerated, this will last up to about 4 weeks, maybe longer. Frozen will last a lot longer. However, if you want to make it shelf stable for up to a year, add ¼ cup of alcohol for every 1 cup of syrup. You can feel free to use brandy or vodka. I would refrigerate this elixir unless you properly can the jars.

Fire Cider
Fire Cider is an immune boosting tonic made with fresh fiery ingredients sure to help your body fight off infections before they begin. This may also put hair on your chest so be forewarned! Once again, this tonic can be consumed daily in one ounce dosages (a shot). If you're fighting illness, take two shots per day.

You'll need a glass quart mason jar to make this. It will also take about 6 weeks to be ready. Feel free to make as much as you want! This is a VERY shelf stable tonic and will not need refrigeration.

- ½ cup each of fresh, grated Ginger and Horseradish 1 whole Lemon diced WITH peel (large)
- 1 medium Onion diced (I used yellow)
- 10 cloves of garlic (you can cut them, mince them or just crush them) 2 large diced Jalapeno Pepper
- 1 TBSP Black Peppercorn
- 1 TBSP Organic Turmeric Powder
- ¼ tsp Organic Cayenne Pepper
- Apple Cider Vinegar
- Dried Rosemary if you have and want to!
- Parchment Paper Cheesecloth
- Raw Honey

Make sure that you grate your Horseradish OUTSIDE or in a well ventilated room. Wear eye covering if you have them! Grating Horseradish can make your eyes and breathing very uncomfortable!

Once you have everything prepped and ready, combine ingredients in your Mason Jar. Add your ACV almost to the very top. I always close the jar and shake it a bit to see if I have added enough vinegar. Do this until you think you have enough.

⇒ Take a piece of parchment and place it on top of the jar and then seal it with the lid. This protects the lid from the vinegar.

⇒ Store in a cool dark cupboard.

⇒ Over the next 4 to 6 weeks, I prefer a full 6 weeks, you will take it out and shake it up. This just makes sure all of the ingredients fully integrate.

⇒ At the end of 6 weeks, strain the liquid with a metal strainer. Then use the cheesecloth to thoroughly squeeze every last drop of your tonic into your Mason Jar.

This is when you add your raw honey to taste. This concoction without the honey WILL be spicy and you don't HAVE to add honey at all. However, the honey may make it not only more palatable but also lends its own antiviral properties to your cider!

Immunity Tea Blend
This tea blend can support your immune system all season long. Herbal teas are easiest to prepare in advance and will last a long time in an airtight glass jar. I love my teas and usually use them at the first hint of viral symptoms. Often, I will brew a cup of this tea if I've been around someone with a cold or virus.

- Equal Parts (¼ cup is a reasonable place to start) Mullein, Dried Elderberries, Peppermint, Dandelion, Echinacea.

Thoroughly blend and seal in an airtight glass container.

⇒ For preventative, steep 1-2 tsp per 8 oz of very hot water, once per day.

⇒ For symptomatic illness, steep 1-2 tsp per 8oz of very hot water 3 times per day.

Fermented Honey Garlic/Ginger
I am of the opinion that everyone should consume at least one clove of garlic per day. You can eat it raw but it could bother your stomach so two other ways to access the pure magic of garlic is to roast it or to make a fermented honey garlic. The fermentation process will soften the garlic and while it is still quite potent, the honey and ginger help take away the worst of the zing of raw garlic. Garlic is SO good for you and everyone should be eating it.

The beauty of Fermented Honey Garlic is that it's an amped up anti EVERYTHING—viral, bacterial, microbial. You can use this on wounds. You can take this for coughs and respiratory illness, or just a teaspoon a day as a preventative. This concoction is also great for cooking so feel free to incorporate it into your kitchen cupboard! Everyone should make this and have it in their cupboard for medicine, culinary use, and just because it's so damn good!

- Garlic
- Ginger
- Raw Honey
- Mason Jar

⇒ Peel your garlic (and ginger if you want to add that!) and lightly crush your garlic to release its juice. This will be what starts the fermentation in the honey!

⇒ Make sure you peel enough to fill whatever size Mason Jar about 2/3 to 3/4 of the way.

Make sure you have RAW honey, preferably local, but definitely RAW from a trusted source, and that is NOT your local supermarket brand. You want unpasteurized and TRUE honey with no corn syrup fillers. If you don't use raw honey it won't ferment and that's a big part of the process!

⇒ Pour your honey over the garlic (and ginger) until it is all submerged but still some room at the top!

⇒ Seal it with your lid. Keep it in a dark, room-temperature place.

I kept mine going for about 2 months but you can use it sooner than that! 4 weeks should do it, the fermentation process will be evidenced by the bubbles that will start.

⇒ Give your honey jar a little upside-down shake every day or so just to keep the garlic covered. Also, it's normal if the jar leaks. It's from the pressure of fermentation! (Dosage per day- 1 Tsp preventative, 3 Tsp active illness)

Summary

I like to be prepared for the cold and flu season and I found that mid to late summer is the best time to begin making these recipes. This way, my family and friends aren't stuck taking over-the-counter meds that really only suppress symptoms and don't truly support their immune system.

Of course, it's important that you understand your body. If you suffer from autoimmune disease it's important to research any and all herbal ingredients. Many of these ingredients don't sit will with autoimmune disease because they will activate an immune response which can work against someone with autoimmune disease. I suffer from an autoimmune disorder and I have catered these recipes to my body. For example, I don't take elderberry daily as a prevention except in the case of direct exposure or if I'm actively symptomatic. I learned that my immune system does not overreact when I do this. The same goes for dandelion. If I take too much dandelion, my immune system overreacts and it can take weeks to recover. So I use dandelion only when I'm sick. I do NOT use echinacea in the immunity tea for my own use but I do for the rest of my family. I cannot stress enough that you need to be responsible for your body.

That being said, remember that this is not medical advice. I am not a doctor. I can only share what I do for me and my family and friends and help you navigate your own experience. Treat all herbs the way you would treat any medication. Many people make the incorrect assumption that just because something is natural, it's good for them. This is not always the case and you should be vigilant by doing research making the best decision about herbal consumption based on that research.

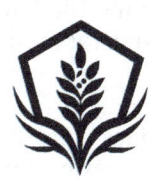

BowTied Mrs Garden *also known as Erin Barone, is a busy but happy wife, mama, grandmama, and Life Coach. She is passionate about helping you navigate your life path in the most holistically healthy way possible! She meets you where you are in whatever journey you are on, offering the time and support you need as you discover new and better ways to live a life full of purpose.*

You can follow her on Twitter at:
@BTMrsGarden

And her website at:
https://coachandclarity.com

ISSUE 2 — SUMMER 2023

The Principles of Regenerative Agriculture

Ryan Griggs

WE are told to find a great family doctor, dentist, this, and that. But we are never told to find a local farmer/rancher that we can trust to provide high quality food. Before diving in, I want to briefly cover regenerative agriculture, a fast-growing sector of agriculture and resources if you want to learn more.

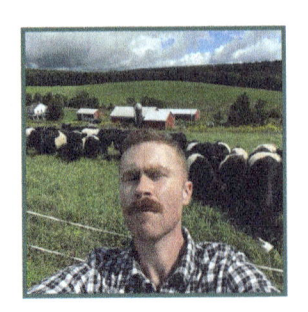

Simply put, regenerative agriculture is aligning with how nature operates, rather than against it (conventional farming). It's not a one size fits all practice; rather, you must understand the land you own along with nature and weather.

There are key principles that are normally practiced in regenerative agriculture such as:

⇒ Minimal tillage. Tilling the land disturbs and kills the microbiology underground, thus destroying topsoil.

⇒ Zero use of herbicides / pesticides / insecticides / fungicides. These toxic chemicals destroy microbiology underground and biodiversity above ground, deplete nutrients in the crops, worsen our health, and to make matters worse, they don't really work. Pests, fungi, and so on build resilience towards chemical sprays.

⇒ Adding crop diversity. Monocropping is a major issue in the US. Drive anywhere in the Midwest and all you see are cornfields. Go to any forest in the world, do you ever see just one species of plant? No, because that's now how nature works. Monocropping depletes the soil & since there isn't biodiversity, any small pest or fungi can ruin everything. What happens then? Spray chemicals, worsening the environment.

⇒ Integrate livestock. Livestock eat the plants and grass and in return nourish the soil with their nutrient-rich manure, which boosts microbial activity underground & protects the soil.

Hands-On Experience
Visit farmers markets and converse with the farmers/ranchers. Show your interest, ask questions about their operation, and want to visit/volunteer. You learn so much just by doing and observing.

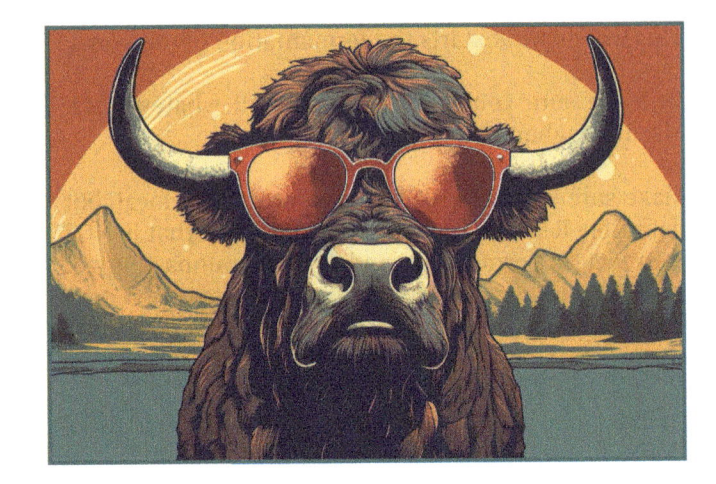

Some resources for hands-on experiences are:

⇒ WWOOF. World Wide Opportunities on Organic Farms. It is not paid, however, you get housing & food in exchange for your labor. It can be a day, weekend, a week, or for me, it was 2-3+ months at a time.

⇒ Quivira Coalition. They have apprenticeships where you are placed with a mentor and work over an 8-month period.

⇒ Greg Judy Grazing School. I have heard nothing but great things about Greg Judy's program. He teaches how to work with livestock and rebuild your soil.

Lastly, utilize your search engine. There are so many programs, farms, and ranches out there looking for folks. ~1% of Americans work in agriculture, they need all the help they can get.

Questions to Ask Your Farmer/Rancher
It's imperative you ask questions in order to really understand who you want to buy your meat and produce from. I have included a list of questions that are handy to ask.

General Questions about the owner:
- How big is their property
- Why they are a farmer / rancher in the first place
- How long have they been a farmer / rancher
- What do they love most about farming / ranching

Questions about animals:
- How frequently do they move their animals to a new pasture / paddock
- What is the herd size
- What common problems do their animals face
- Do they use antibiotics & hormones for their animals
- What supplements do you give your animals if any
- What do they feed their animals with
- Are the animals ever confined, if so why?
- How do they care for the animals, especially in the wintertime. What is their winter feed?
- What breed are the animals & why
- Do they process USDA or local / state
- Age of slaughter

Questions about their crops:
- What variety of crops do they grow & how do they grow them
- Do they spray any herbicides / pesticides / insecticides? (produce NOT sprayed is higher in antioxidants, more nutritious, and lower in toxic heavy metals.)
- What is the harvest date of their crops
- How do they keep their crops healthy
- Do they do any type of soil testing

Above all else, you should visit the farm/ranch & see everything for yourself. If they do not allow visitors, that is usually a bad sign. More often than not, farmers/ranchers would love to have you visit & see their operation. Lastly, there are a couple other ways to meet your farmer/rancher outside directly calling/visiting them.

Farmers markets are a great way to develop relationships with your local farmers/ranchers. Show your interest, ask questions about their operation, and want to visit/volunteer. You learn so much just by doing and observing.

https://www.usdalocalfoodportal.com/ is a great resource to find nearby farmers markets.

Regenerative Agriculture Resources

Documentaries:
- To Which We Belong
- Biggest Little Farm
- Burned the Movie
- Kiss the Ground
- Farmer's Footprint
- A Life on Our Planet: My Witness Statement
- Fantastic Fungi
- Honeyland
- The Pollinators Before the Plate Sacred Cow

Books:
- Dirt to Soil
- City Chicks
- Defending Beef
- The CAFO Reader
- Holistic Management 3rd Edition
- The Unsettling of America
- Sacred Cow
- Cows Save the Planet
- The Soil Will Save Us
- Grass, Soil, Hope
- Growing a Revolution
- For the Love of Soil
- Call of the Reed Warbler
- Any Joel Salatin

YouTube:
- Allan Savory
- Joel Salatin
- Gabe Brown
- Greg Judy
- Kiss the Ground
- Savory Institute
- Search regenerative agriculture—there are so many amazing accounts showing their day-to-day work, explaining different methods, diving into the business aspects, etc.

Podcasts:
- Meat Mafia
- Down to Earth
- Ground Work
- Regeneration Rising
- The Thriving Farmer Podcast
- Joe Rogan: Joel Salatin, Will Harris episodes
- TFTC episode 243—Regenerative farming with Untapped Growth (on Twitter)

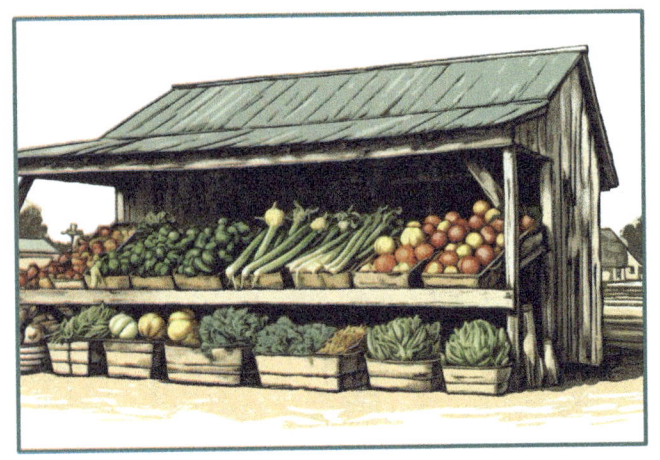

Consider joining a CSA or Community-Supported Agriculture. Joining a CSA is essentially a membership with the farmer where you get produce directly from them weekly. It can also vary from farm to farm. For example, the farm I worked on that had a CSA ran it a bit differently. The customer would give them a lump sum at the beginning of the year and in exchange get the farmer's produce and meats at a discounted rate. Every Wednesday was CSA day where folks could visit the farm and buy directly at the barn. It was a great way to see the relationships between the farmer and customers. Local harvest is a great resource to find a local CSA. https://www.localharvest.org/csa/

Ryan Griggs *made a switch from working in tech (IBM) to becoming a regenerative rancher. He is founder and CEO of* The Regenaissance, *an apparel-based brand reconnecting us back to where our food is grown and promoting the regeneration of our health through diet, exercise, and the outdoors.*

You can follow him on Twitter at:
@_ryan_griggs

And see his Website at:
https://theregenaissance.co

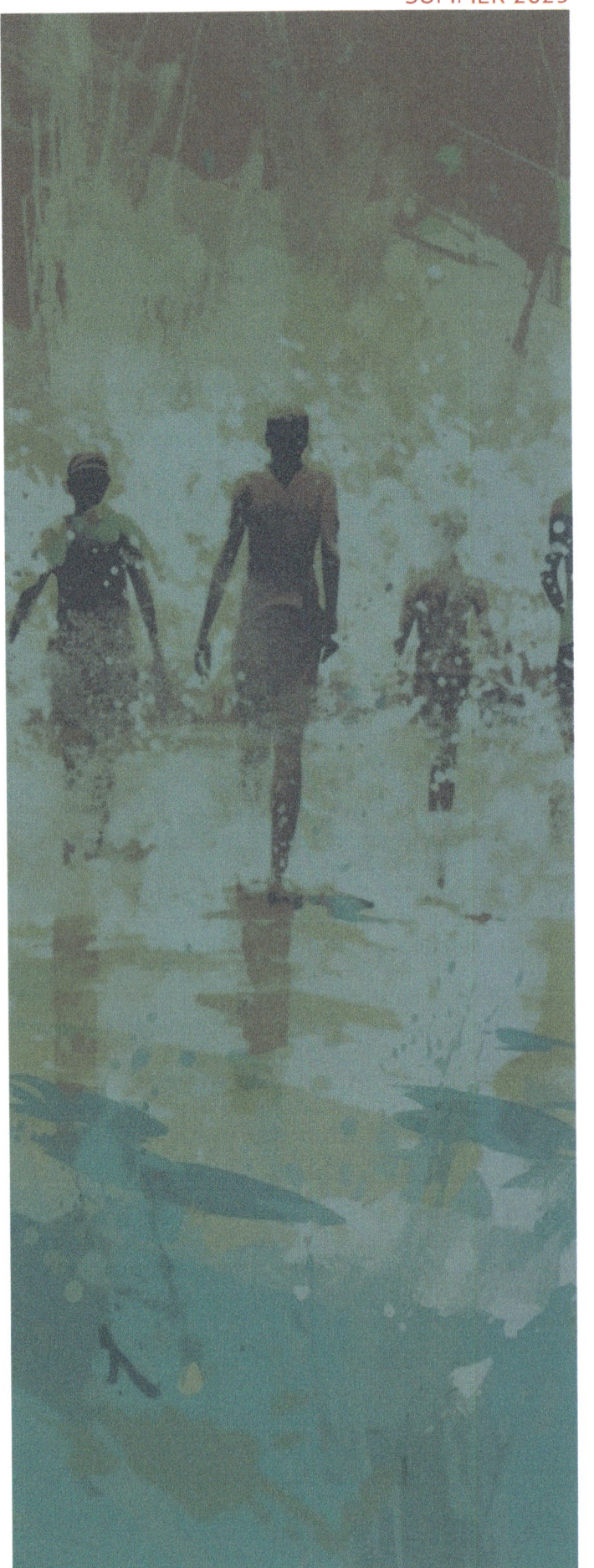

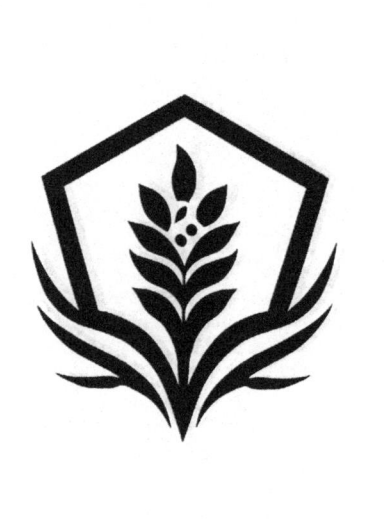

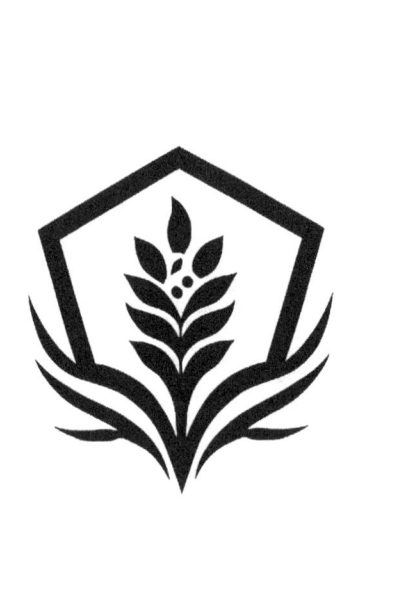

Made in the USA
Monee, IL
24 October 2023